A Child Is Born

Lennart Nilsson

Text by **Lars Hamberger**

A Merloyd Lawrence Book

Delacorte Press/Seymour Lawrence

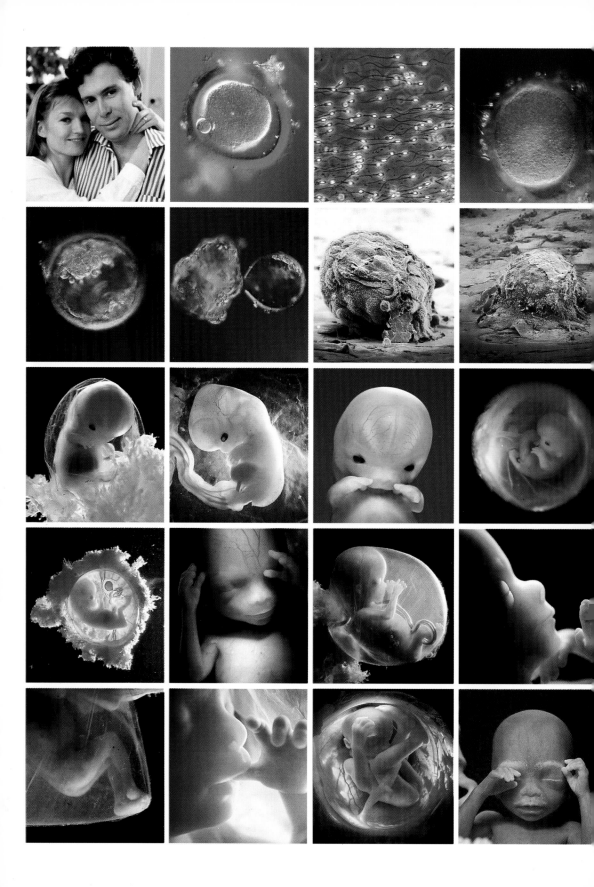

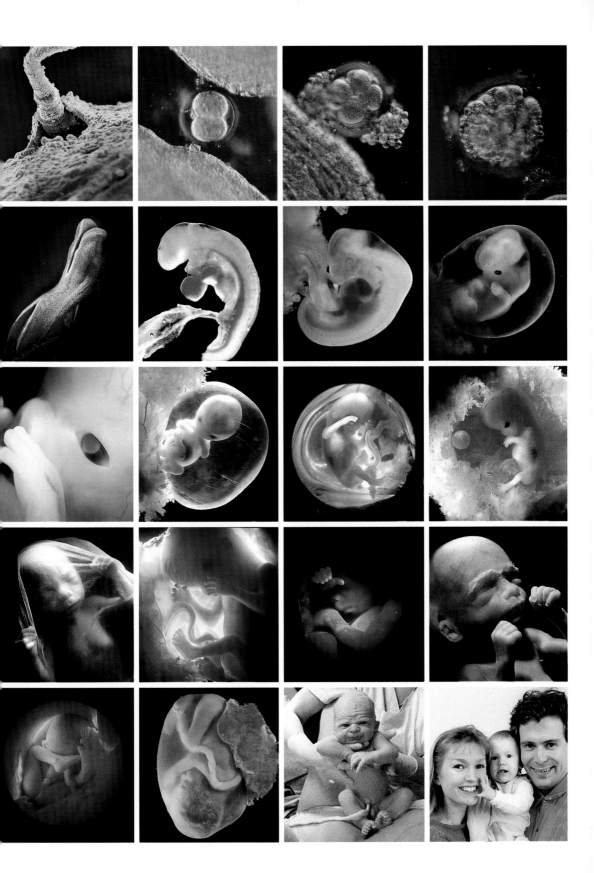

Translated into English by Clare James

Editor Per Wivall
Design and color drawings Bo Berling
Assistant Catharina Fjellström-Nilsson
Coloring of scanning electron photos Gillis Häägg
Typesetting Ytterlids, Falkenberg
Lithography Repronik, Mölndal
Printed and bound by Arnoldo Mondadori S.p.A., Verona 1990

Published by
Delacorte Press/Seymour Lawrence
Bantam Doubleday Dell Publishing Group, Inc.
666 Fifth Avenue
New York, New York 10103

Originally published in Sweden under the title *Ett barn blir till* by Albert Bonniers Förlag, Stockholm.
Completely new edition copyright © 1990 Lennart Nilsson Photography AB, In Vitro AB, and Bonnier Fakta AB.
English translation copyright © 1990 by Bantam Doubleday Dell Publishing Group, Inc.

Library of Congress Cataloging-in-Publication Data

Nilsson, Lennart 1922-
[Ett barn blir till. English]
A child is born/Lennart Nilsson. — Completely new ed./ text by Lars Hamberger.
p. cm.
Translation of: Ett barn blir till
"A Merloyd Lawrence book."
Includes bibliographical references.
   ISBN 0-385-30237-1 $ 25.00
   1. Pregnancy.   2. Childbirth.   3. Pregnancy — pictorial works
4. Childbirth — Pictorial works.   I. Hamberger, Lars.   II. Title
RG525.N5413 1990
612.6'3'0222 — dc20   90-33633
                                                                        CIP

Manufactured in Italy
Published simultaneously in Canada

October 1990

10 9 8 7 6 5 4 3 2

Contents

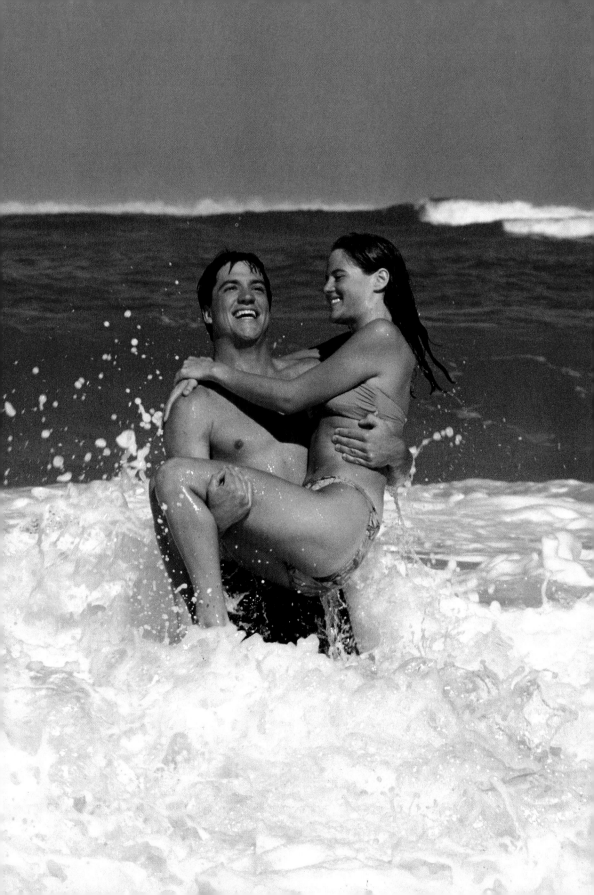

In the Beginning

From generation to generation, life renews itself in the encounter between male and female. Billions of years ago, this meeting took place in the sea, where creatures of both sexes shed their reproductive cells into the surrounding water. Eventually terrestrial animals were able to range far over the earth because they carried the salty ocean environment within themselves, whether inside the female body or inside a protective eggshell. The sea, as the original nursery of life, still remains a powerful natural attraction for human beings, a source of exhilaration and renewal.

While life has found ever more diverse ways to reproduce itself, almost every new creature, whether a human baby or a sea urchin, begins with a single cell. Within this one cell, the fertilized ovum or egg cell, which contains genes from both male and female, is the entire genetic code of the future individual. Through each one of us, the intricate blueprint is passed on to posterity. This powerful system, evolved over billions of years, ensures that human beings will give birth to human beings, whales to whales, and hummingbirds to hummingbirds. At the

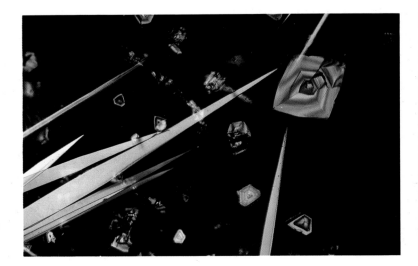

Billons of years ago the first living organisms appeared in the sea. Even today, all land animals, including human beings, carry this original watery environment within themselves.
Right, sex hormones in their crystalline form. The man's testosterone is stiletto-sharp, while the woman's estrogen is a broader shape known as rhomboid.

same time, it makes diversity possible. Except for identical twins, no one individual is just like any other, and mutations over the centuries allow each species to evolve.

The energies which bring men and women together still link us with all other living creatures. We respond to deep biological forces of which we are hardly aware. For instance, like many other members of the animal kingdom, we are strongly influenced by erotic stimulants called *pheremones*, chemical stimulants secreted by each sex.

Human reproduction, a relatively new stage in the history of life on earth, introduces a new element in the courtship and mating of males and females: that of conscious choice. Among mammals, human sexual maturity comes relatively late; attraction and bonding are complicated. Personal preference, cultural values, the rules imposed by various religions – all these influence not only the relationships between men and women but the way women give birth around the world. In modern times even politics has entered the picture, as some governments attempt to enforce pro-birth policies while others respond to the ever more serious threat of overpopulation.

Young couples contemplating parenthood today ask themselves many thoughtful and important questions: What kind of world will we bring our baby into? What does a child deserve from us – a healthy start, education, economic security, a home with both a mother and a father, with a brother or sister? Answers to these questions will vary from couple to couple, from one country, one religon, one culture to another. In many

Powerful signals

Although our sense of smell is inferior to that of most animals, human beings, like other species, have been found to secrete chemical "lures," substances called *pheremones*. The concentration of these varies, rising during a kiss, for example.

Right, pheremone molecules magnified 400,000 times. The organs targeted by these erotic stimulants, and their precise effects, still elude scientific investigators.

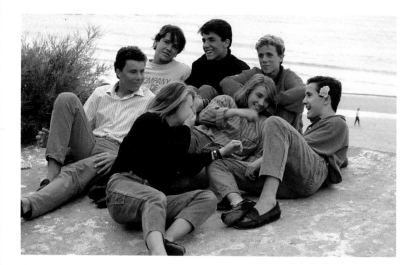

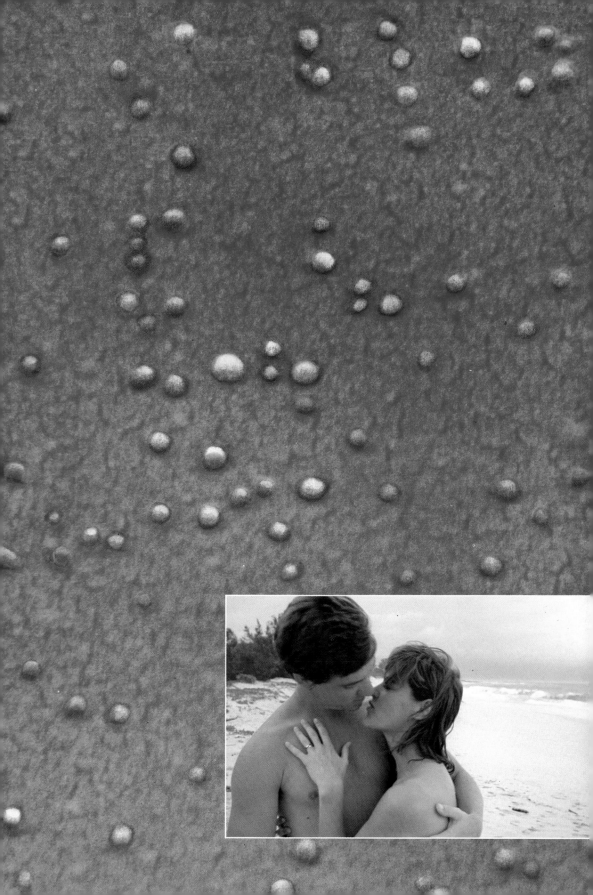

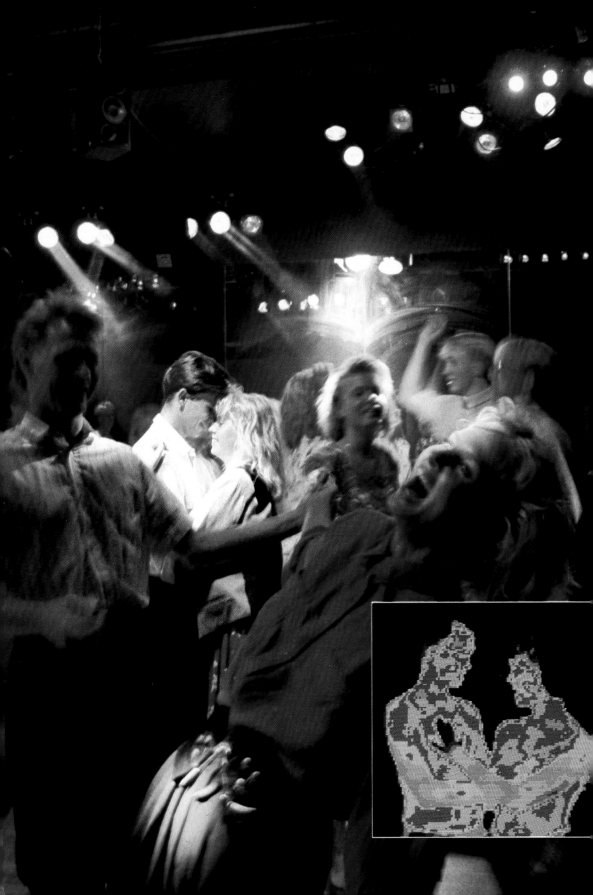

respects the answers today can be more optimistic. In general, birth is safer for both mother and baby than ever before. The life expectancy of a child born today is longer than ever before. Though poverty still afflicts millions of children, the very questions that conscientious couples now ask before plunging into parenthood may lead us to provide a cleaner, safer, more loving world for later generations. Now, as childbirth becomes safer and more babies grow to adulthood, our greatest responsibility is to leave our children and grandchildren a healthy and unspoiled planet.

The more scientists have learned about the beginning of human life, the greater the wonder has become. In this book we try to portray in words, and above all in pictures, the story of the nine months from ovulation to birth. New technology has made it possible to see the actual events surrounding fertilization and to visualize the growing fetus more clearly. At the same time, new medical knowledge has reduced the risks of pregnancy and has given couples greater choice as to how their child will be born. Recent scientific advances enable us to take better care of babies born too early, and also to help couples who have trouble conceiving. We have tried to reflect this new knowledge and these recent advances throughout the chapters of our book.

At the center of our story, however, is neither technology nor modern medicine but the enduring miracle of pregnancy and birth. We hope both to illuminate and to celebrate this universal experience.

A kiss – as seen by a thermocamera

A thermocamera measures differences in temperature between various skin areas: blue is cool and red is warm. In the middle picture we can see the temperature in the woman's chest rise.

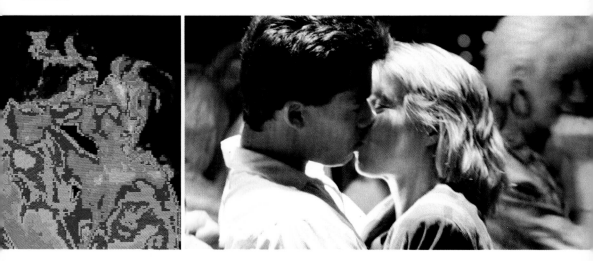

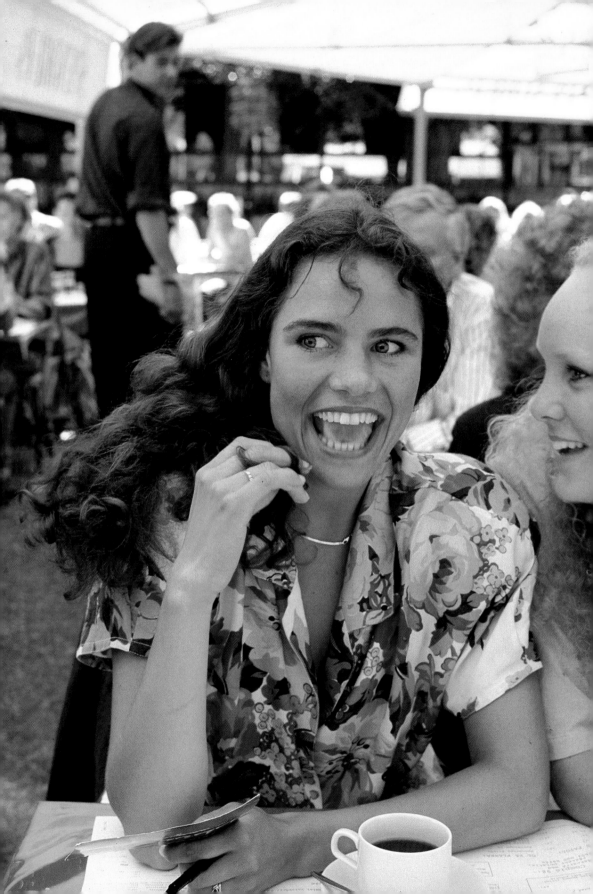

The Woman

For each of us, gender has been determined since egg and sperm fused, at the very moment of fertilization. Sperm carry the genetic blueprint for gender. Both external and internal sex organs take shape early in pregnancy and by the fifth month all the eggs a woman will ever produce (some five million) have already formed in the fetal ovaries. If the sex organs of the female fetus are exposed to some toxic substance or infection during this period, this may not be detected until much later in life, when the adult woman consults a doctor for menstrual disorders or failure to conceive.

The growing girl differs both physically and mentally from the boy, long before the onset of sexual maturity. To a schoolteacher, this is abundantly clear. Teachers know that, in the early school years, girls generally show greater readiness for school, learn to read faster and often regard the childish and immature boys in the class with a certain indulgence. This lead often persists well into the teenage years. At the age of 11 or 12, the onset of female sexual maturity takes the form of a spurt in growth, swelling breasts and an increasingly womanly distribution of body hair. Soon menstruation begins as well.

Why do certain people take a fancy to each other, while others leave one another cold? There are no easy answers. A smile, a second glance, a brief encounter—attraction is highly unpredictable.

Estrogen, the female sex hormone—*right*, in crystalline form—is a signal that, via the bloodstream, reaches all kinds of tissue, giving the woman's body its specific characteristics.

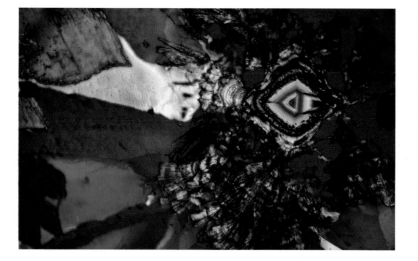

17

A century ago, young girls in Western Europe and the U.S. did not begin menstruating until the age of 15 or 16. Today, the first menstruation, or menarche, occurs much earlier. This change came about because of our increasingly nutritious diet, since it is weight—rather than age—that determines the timing of the menarche. The proportion of body fat seems to be a factor, for menstruation is often delayed for young female athletes in training.

Each menstrual period initiates a cycle which is on average four weeks, but may range from three to five weeks. The first signals in this cycle are emitted by the pituitary gland, a tiny hormone-producing organ located at the base of the brain. Centers in the lower portions of the brain directly connected with the pituitary gland determine which hormones are secreted. Menstruation may be delayed or cease entirely if a woman experiences grief and anxiety, is severely ill or under heavy pressure at work. But even minor changes in a woman's life can affect her menstrual periods—a holiday trip, for example, or the desire to become pregnant.

If the woman's mental state is more or less in equilibrium, the brain permits the pituitary gland to secrete special hormones that are conducted to the ovaries in the bloodstream. The ovaries respond to this stimulation by increasing their production of the female sex hormone estrogen. Simultaneously, an ovum (egg) starts to ripen in one of the ovaries. This will lead to ovulation: the release of the ovum from the capsule-like structure which contains it, known as the *follicle*.

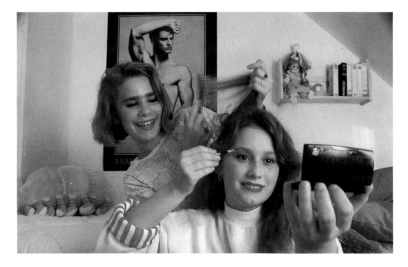

Girlhood begins to give way to womanhood. The toys in a teenage girl's room give way to posters, tapes and novels. Meanwhile, remarkable developments are taking place within the girl's body, and its contours are becoming typically female. These changes can create an intense interest in her physical appearance.

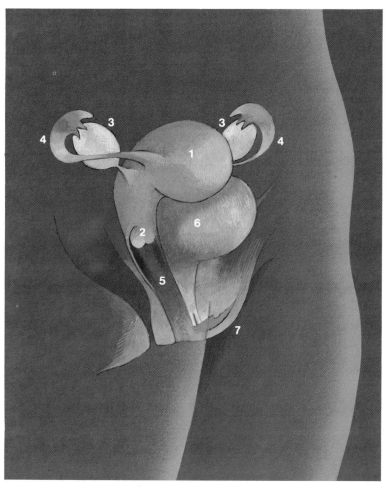

A woman's monthly cycle is governed by the interplay of hormones between certain parts of the brain on the one hand and the ovaries on the other. The lower part of the brain (hypothalamus) stimulates the pituitary gland, causing it to release gonadotropic hormones (*blue arrow*), which reach the ovaries via the bloodstream. The ovaries respond by producing steroid hormones; these, too, circulate in the blood, acting on the pituitary gland to inhibit its hormone production (*red arrow*). This feedback process is repeated each month.

(1) uterus, (2) cervix, (3) ovary, (4) Fallopian tube, (5) vagina, (6) bladder, (7) labia minora and labia majora

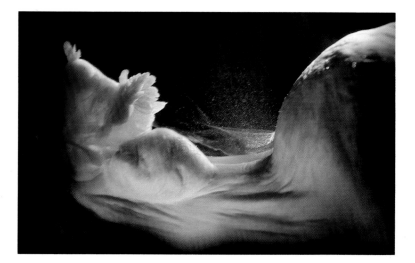

Right, the fimbriae of the Fallopian tube have just begun the search for a ripe follicle ready to rupture on the ovarian surface (in the middle of the picture). The womb is sharply outlined to the right.

Interplay of female hormones

A woman often notices that ovulation is approaching, since her vaginal mucus becomes more copious. The mucus comes from the uterus (womb) and the cervix (neck of the womb), and at the time of ovulation it becomes more abundant, transparent and capable of forming a thread. It is only when the cervical mucus has these properties that the sperm can pass through it into the uterus. Daily observations of these changes in the cervical secretions are used in a contraceptive technique known as *natural family planning*. In this method, which is as yet far from foolproof because of variations in the menstrual cycle, sexual intercourse is avoided for several days before and after ovulation. The same observations may also, of course, be used when the woman is trying to conceive, to determine the day in the menstrual cycle on which fertility is greatest.

Two weeks after the onset of the menstrual period, the follicle containing the ovum is ripe. It measures roughly 2 cm (about .8 inch) in diameter and, as well as serving as a container for the ovum, has also itself become a tiny hormone-producing gland. Suddenly the follicle ruptures—exactly why is as yet unknown. The ovum is now discharged to the surface of the ovary, where it is caught up by the Fallopian tube. For about 24 hours, it awaits possible fertilization by a sperm; if this does not occur the ovum begins to disintegrate and dies.

Once the follicle has ruptured, it is transformed into a structure known as the corpus luteum, which forms large quantities of progesterone for the next two weeks. The progesterone enters the woman's bloodstream, making changes throughout her body, in particular altering the endometrium, the lining of the uterus, preparing it to receive a fertilized ovum. Thus, the

Gateway to life

The cervix protrudes into the upper part of the vagina. The opening of the cervix leads into the uterus. When ovulation occurs, transparent cervical mucus issues from this opening. The mucus screens out the sperm— making a preliminary selection—when sexual intercourse takes place. After only a day or so, the cervix closes. For the remainder of the menstrual cycle, a viscous plug of mucus prevents the passage into the uterus of even the most vigorous sperm. Through this gateway to life, the baby will also pass during delivery.

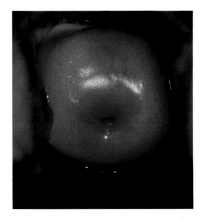

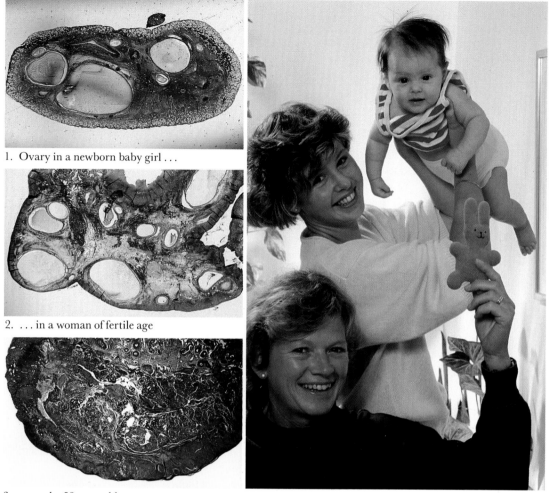

1. Ovary in a newborn baby girl . . .

2. . . . in a woman of fertile age

3. . . . and a 50-year-old woman.

Three generations of women — and their ovaries. Even in the newborn baby girl, each ovary contains many almost-ripe ovum cells (1). Nature is not stingy; there are plenty of ova for the approximately 400 ovulations that are to take place during the woman's fertile years. In the mother — generation two — the ovaries are replete with ova at various stages of maturity (2). In the grandmother, the ovaries' task is accomplished: now, no more ova ripen and the ovaries shrivel (3).

uterus is prepared for pregnancy every month. If this does not happen, the outer layers of the endometrium are shed, causing the superficial capillary damage and the bleeding that we call menstruation.

Menstruation can be seen as the final phase in a series of hormonal changes that take place in the woman's body each month — repeating themselves, broadly speaking, from the menarche in the early teenage years until the last menstrual period, at the time of the menopause when the woman is about 50. All together, the woman menstruates roughly 400 times. The menopause, or "change of life" as it is sometimes called, is often blamed for a series of problems, such as tiredness, difficulties in concentrating, insomnia, hot flashes (flushes) and a great deal else. For many women, however, the cessation of menstruation entails no such symptoms.

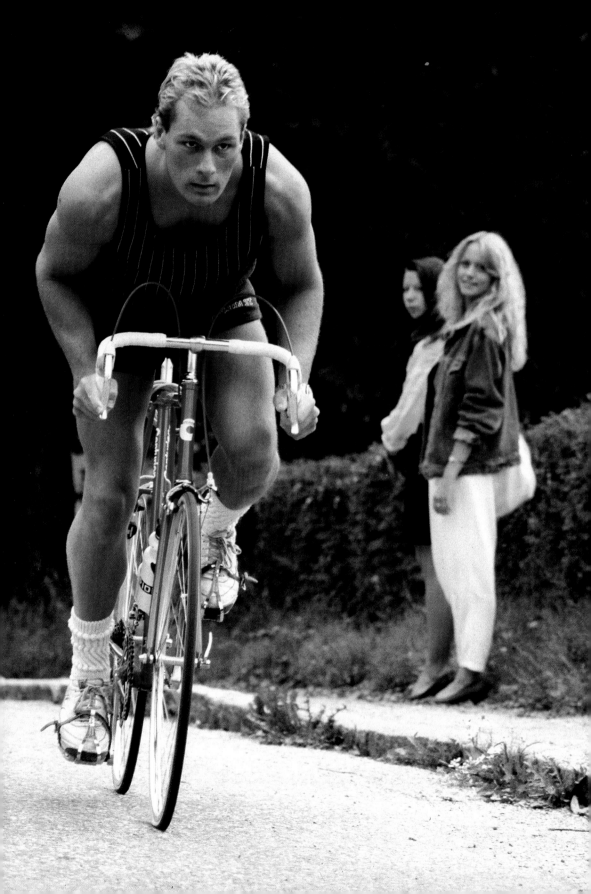

The Man

Though the story of Genesis tells us that the first human being was a man, knowledge of biology shows that both men and women must have appeared on Earth simultaneously. When all forms of life existed in the sea, both male and female sex cells were released into the ocean environment where they fused and grew. Certain marine species still reproduce this way, but in creatures leaving the sea for a terrestrial life, the male and the female roles became sharply differentiated.

Each of us—male as well as female—started as an embryo, programmed and developed from the genetic blueprint in a sperm with the male chromosome, Y, and an ovum with the X chromosome. Chromosomes are the bodies within a nucleus which bear the genes. Although genetic information differs greatly between men and women, it is very hard to see any external difference between boys and girls during the first few months of fetal development. Later, in a male fetus, the testes descend from a position inside the abdominal cavity into the scrotum. Sometimes the testes fail to descend and a minor operation to "pull" them down into the scrotum may be necessary. In general, like many animals, men are capable of drawing their testes up toward the abdominal cavity in hazardous situations; this is one of the special design features created by nature to safeguard reproduction.

Robust bones and strong muscles are programmed into a man's genes and the male sex hormone, testosterone, stimulates their development. Not all men attain such impressive results as this well-exercised cyclist. But not every woman seeks an athlete for a mate. The image of an ideal male differs from culture to culture and over the years, just as standards of female beauty tend to evolve.

Right, the testosterone crystal, a multicolored kite in the world of hormones.

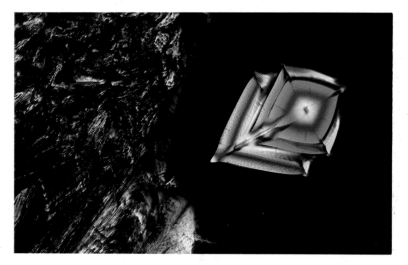

From boy to man

A baby boy at the moment of birth already has numerous immature sperm cells or *spermatogonia*. As in the woman, hormones from the pituitary gland are primarily responsible for male sexual maturation and the initiation of sperm production. The pituitary gland produces exactly the same hormones in both sexes, but its functions are, in turn, regulated by the part of the brain called the hypothalamus, and here there are major differences between the sexes. In men, the hypothalamus contains specific areas that are sensitive to the male sex hormone, known as testosterone.

Why is it, then, that boys do not begin to mature sexually until they are 12 or 13 years old? There is still no clear answer to this question but we do know that the thymus, a secretory gland located in the upper part of the thoracic cavity, has a capacity to delay sexual development. The onset of sexual maturity and puberty in the early teens is caused by two different hormones from the pituitary gland. One helps the testicles to form the male sex hormone testosterone, while the other assists in the production and maturation of sperm.

Growth of the body and the external sex organs, deepening ("breaking") of the voice and the development of hair on the face and body are governed by testosterone. Thus, it is this hormone that makes boys grow taller than girls and their muscles become larger. Testosterone is also required for the sperm to mature and the sex organs to become fully operative.

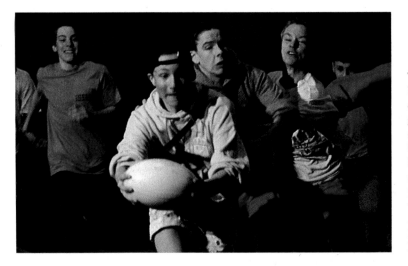

The masculine role has long been associated with an interest in tough, demanding games in which the muscles come into play and aggressive impulses burgeon. This behavior evolved on the savanna around a million years ago, when the man had to defend his family and tribe. A big, strong man still enjoys high status, although we need him less.

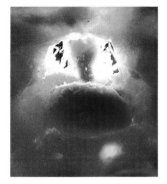

Like a woman's, a man's sex hormone is regulated by the brain and the pituitary gland, a tiny oval body at the base of the skull. Via the bloodstream, their signals reach his testicles, which produce testosterone. Hormone balance is maintained through feedback.

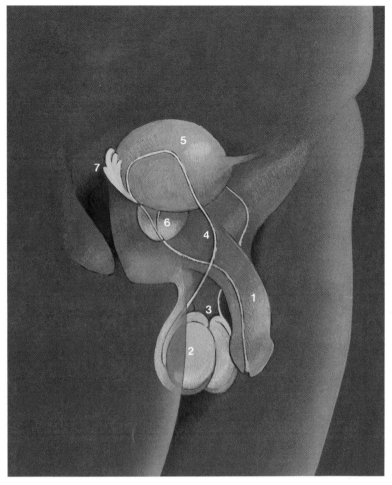

Below, the stiffening penis as registered by a thermocamera. The blue patches show a relatively low temperature, while the red ones are warmer. The *middle* picture shows the incipient erection; *right*, the fully erect penis, of which the end part, the glans, is the warmest.

(1) penis with urethra, (2) testicle, (3)epididymis, (4) vas deferens, (5) bladder, (6) prostate gland, (7) seminal vesicle

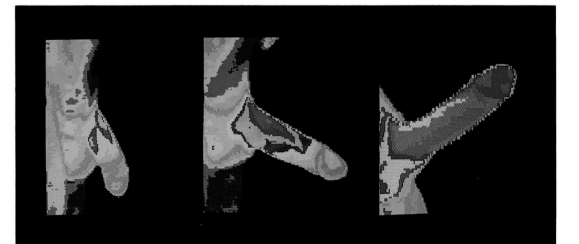

A thousand sperm a second

Sperm production is the most astounding of the human body's phenomenal production systems. Every day, as shown here, a healthy young male body produces nearly 100 million sperm, i.e. 1,000 sperm a second. Each sperm, moreover, contains an entirely unique selection of the father-to-be's genetic material. The sperm are produced in the long, convoluted passageways of the testes known as the seminiferous tubules.

The picture *below* shows a cross section of a seminiferous tubule. In the outermost layer of the tubules, the primitive sperm (spermatogonia) are formed. These take a good two months to mature, and during this time they move inward from the periphery toward the central, open duct. During this migration each spermatogonium divides twice, thus giving rise to four sperm. These are nourished by special cells and pushed, tail first, into the duct (see picture and enlargement, *right*). They are then transported to the epididymis for storage.

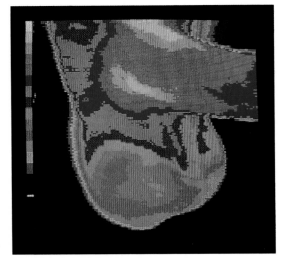

The thermocamera reveals that the temperature in the scrotum is only 35° C (about 95° F), i.e. lower than in the rest of the body—an essential requirement if the sperm is to be capable of fertilization.

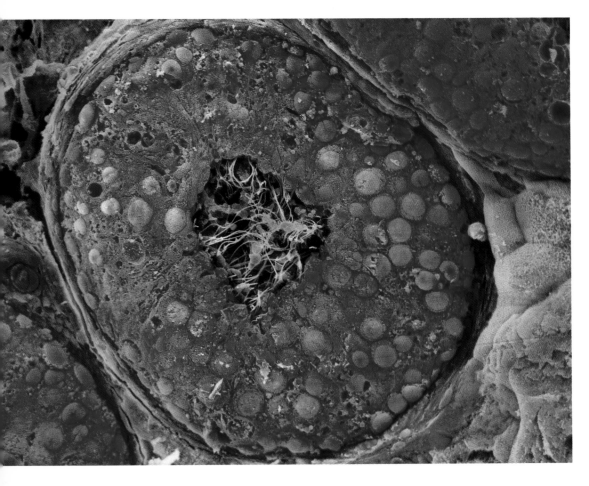

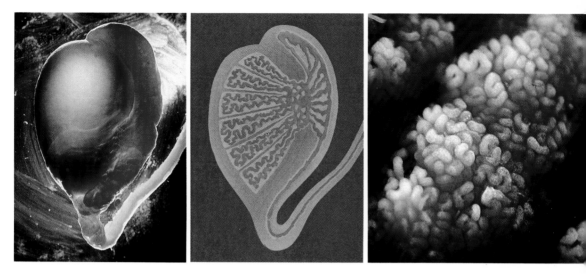

The man's sex gland, the testis, is roughly half the size of an ordinary chicken's egg and linked to the epididymis, where the sperm are stored. The drawing shows, in cross section, how the seminiferous tubules are arranged in compartments. The picture *above* shows the coils of a single tubule. All together, the length of the tubules is several hundred meters.

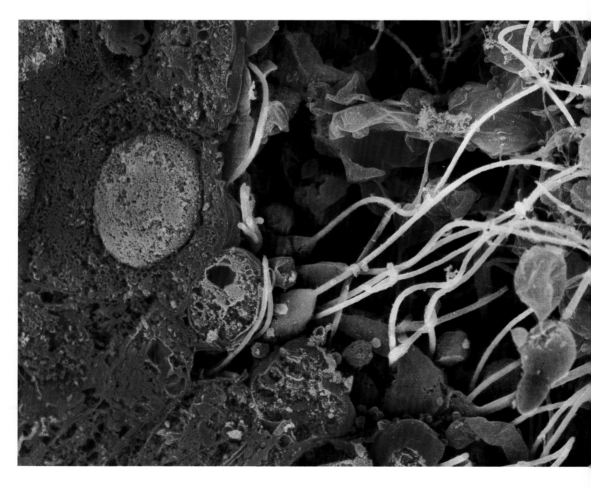

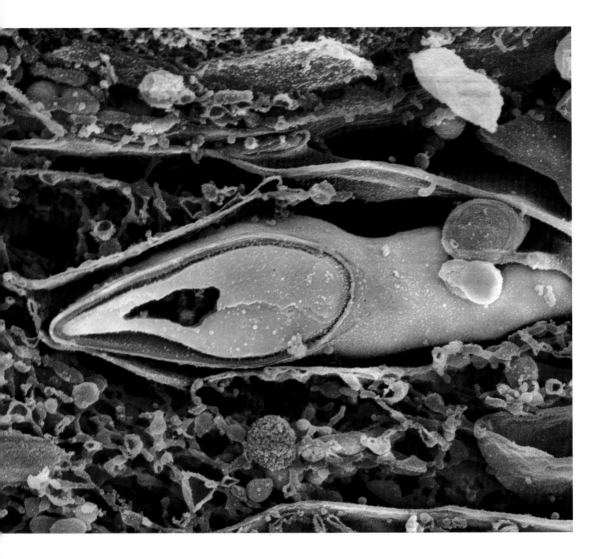

Loaded with genes

The sperm is six-hundredths of a millimeter (about
.00024 inch) long. Here, it is shown with the head in
cross section while still deep inside the testis. The
head contains the man's genetic material, packed
closely together. It is protected by a cap-like structure
or acrosome, which is shown in red in the picture
above. *Right*, the acrosomes of the sperm are illuminated in red by means of fluorescence. The acrosome
contains enzymes that help the sperm to penetrate the
wall of the ovum. The sperm retains its cap until it
approaches the ovum, and then sheds it—possibly
under the influence of substances produced by the
ovum. Thus, a kind of chemical ping-pong is played
between ovum and sperm.

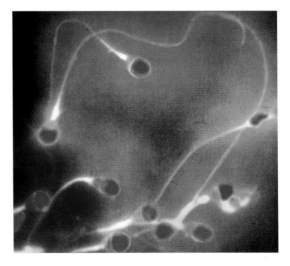

Mass production with numerous rejects

The male body constantly forms new sperm capable of fertilization. This occurs from sexual maturity up to a very advanced age, while a woman's egg cells are formed during the fetal stage, and never again. Men have become fathers in their eighties.

While a woman, in general, develops only one ovum capable of fertilization each month, the man can produce billions of new sperm, each of a unique genetic composition, in the same amount of time. At each ejaculation, 2–5 milliliters (about ½ to just over 1 teaspoon) of seminal fluid containing up to 500 million mobile sperm is discharged. But almost half the sperm of a healthy young man have small defects that prevent them from fertilizing an ovum.

Before ejaculation, sperm have matured and been stored in the epididymis. When sexual excitation culminates in ejaculation, the sperm are thrust at great speed through each vas deferens and into the urethra. There, they are mixed with a secretion from the prostate gland containing substances that facilitate their long journey to the female ovum. The seminal liquid is discharged with immense force by means of contractions of the pelvic muscles: first the sperm and the prostate secretion, followed by a sugar-containing fluid from the seminal vesicles (glands emptying into the vas deferens).

The ability of the penis to swell, stiffen and become erect under the influence of sexual excitement is due to the increased flow of blood through the erectile tissue, which becomes engorged. After ejaculation, the blood supply diminishes and the erectile tissue reverts to its former slack state.

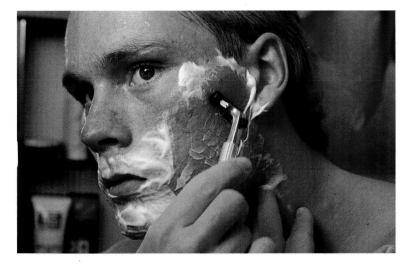

A young man's sprouting beard and the incipient hirsuteness on his chest, arms and legs are caused by the sex hormone testosterone. From its site of production in the testicles, the hormone is distributed in the bloodstream to its target cells, the hair roots. Other effects of testosterone are large muscles and a deep voice.

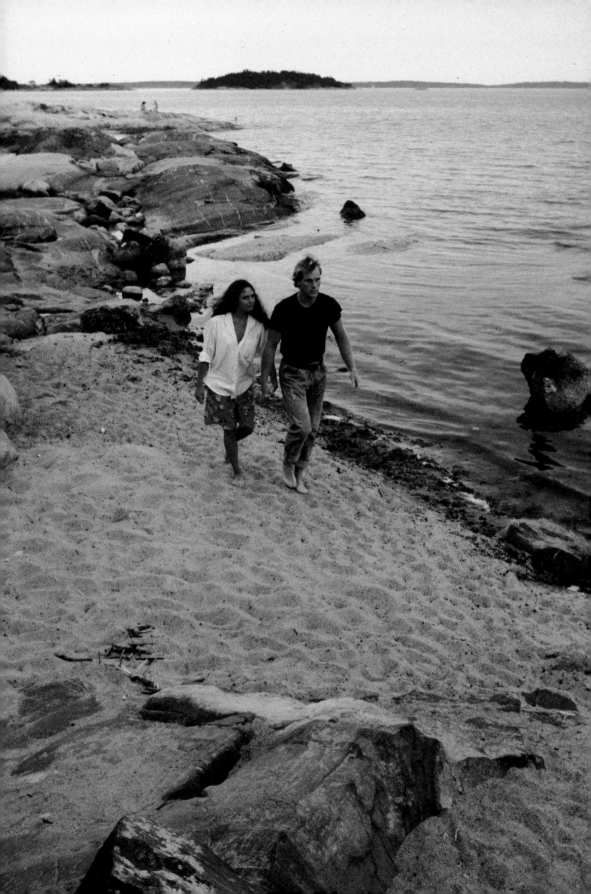

Ovulation

In the course of a woman's life, ovulation occurs about 400 times all together. It is very much a matter of chance which of the two ovaries sheds the ovum; the ovaries do not always take turns. If one ovary is surgically removed for any reason, ovulation will take place each month in the remaining ovary. This seems to be one way in which the body protects itself against diseases of the reproductive organs. However, most of the woman's egg cells are never used. Most of her almost half-million eggs have the same potential to be fertilized, but never fully ripen; instead, they gradually degenerate. By the time the woman ceases to ovulate, at the age of 50 or so, there are no healthy ova left.

Ovulation itself is a dynamic process that takes place in the course of one or more minutes. The portion of the follicle facing the abdominal cavity ruptures fairly rapidly and the fluid (10–15 ml or 2/3 to 1 tablespoon) filling the follicle and containing millions of cells that have produced female sex hormones runs out. In the midst of this vast number of cells is the ovum, the follicle's most valuable cargo. It is surrounded by thousands of cells that provide nourishment and protection for the journey.

A beautiful day by the seaside, endlessly walking along the beach. A man and a woman decide to have a baby.

At ovulation a woman can become pregnant. Here, *right*, ovulation is imminent. A fluid-filled follicle rises from the surface of one ovary. The funnel of the Fallopian tube hovers over the ovary's surface, ready to collect the ovum.

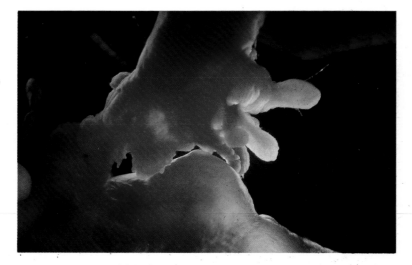

Release and capture of the ovum

Several hours before the actual ovulation, the Fallopian tube has probably received signals as to the site on the ovary's surface where the rupture will take place. The fimbriae (finger-like projections of the Fallopian tube) have positioned themselves to catch the ovum and prevent it from disappearing into the abdominal cavity. The soft folds in the mucous membrane of the fimbriae move unceasingly back and forth across the ovary's surface, apparently tasting the chemical messenger substances there. The entire membrane is covered with tiny cilia, all beating in toward the interior of the Fallopian tube and creating a kind of suction for the fluid shed by the follicle. With this fluid comes further information in the form of chemical signals, making the muscles in the Fallopian tube begin contracting rhythmically. These contractions help the cilia trap the ovum.

Occasionally the Fallopian tube—if it is long and mobile— can reach the opposite ovary. It then begins to compete, trying to draw in the ovum and sometimes actually succeeding in doing so. The fact that ova can "jump across" to the opposite Fallopian tube is known for certain since women have become pregnant despite the absence of a Fallopian tube on one side and an ovary on the other.

The Fallopian tube's mobility may be severely impaired if the woman has ever suffered from an inflammation of the tube caused by, for example, gonorrhea or chlamydia. During the healing process, adhesions form around the Fallopian tube, hindering it from capturing the ovum. At worst, the whole tube becomes blocked so that the woman is unable to conceive.

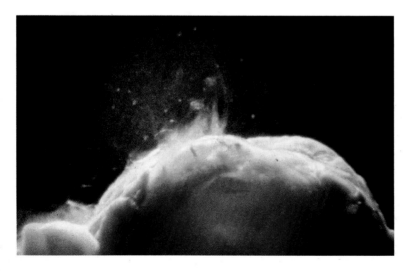

Suddenly the follicle ruptures, ejecting fluid containing thousands of hormone-producing cells—and, in its midst, the ovum, smaller than a pin-head (see *left* and enlargement on *right*). The ovum is surrounded by nutrient cells that give it ample nourishment during its journey to the uterus.

Inserts: *top*, the ovum is about to be sucked into the funnel of the Fallopian tube.

Below, the empty follicle, which often bleeds slightly. Soon the hole is sealed and the follicle transformed into a hormone-producing gland known as the corpus luteum. To the left of the follicle is the end of the Fallopian tube.

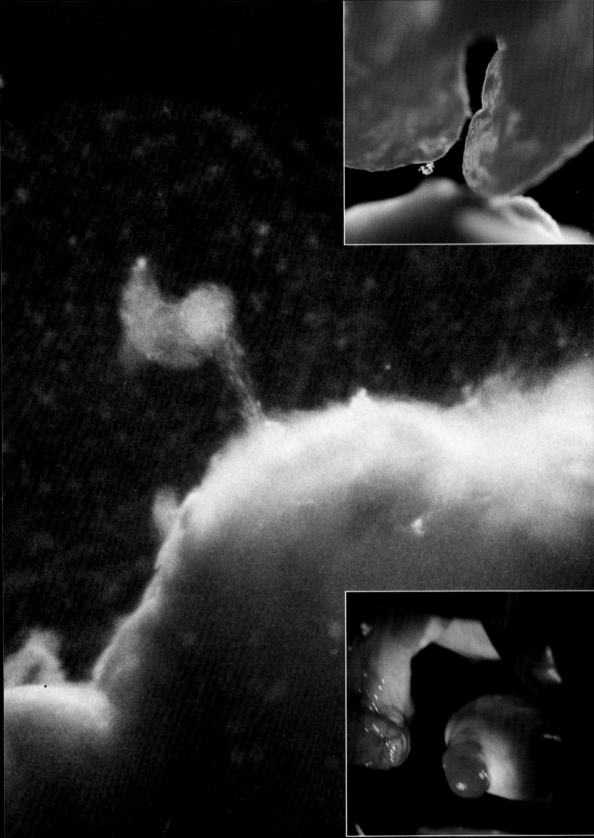

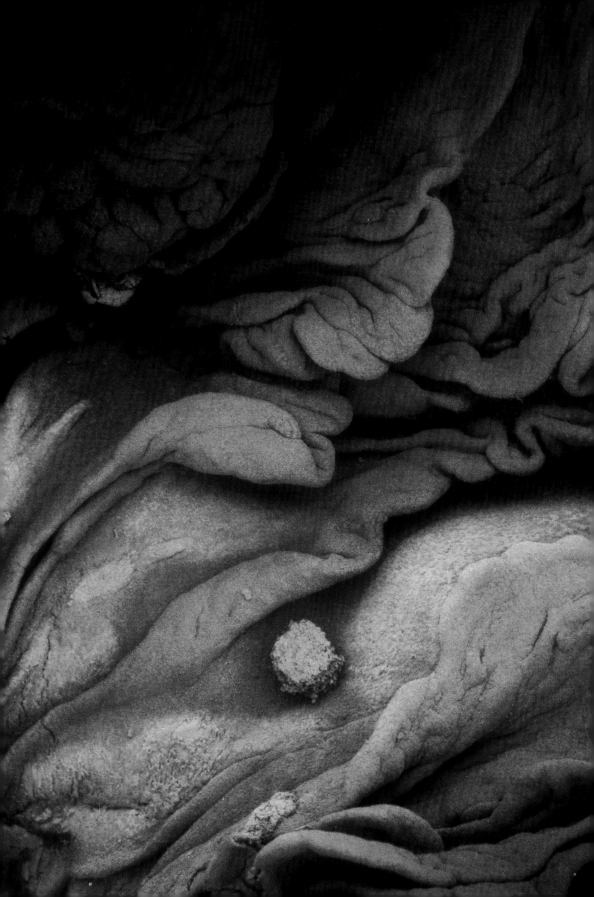

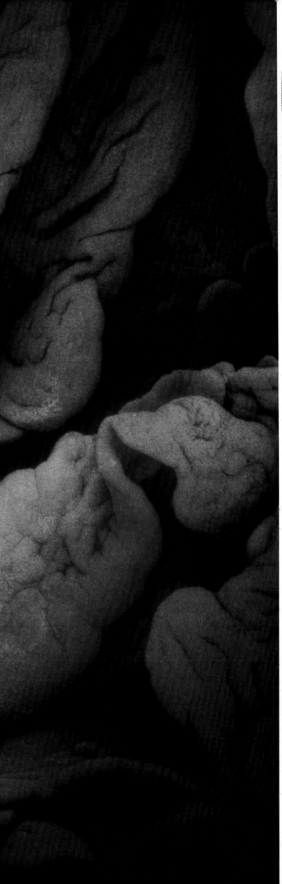

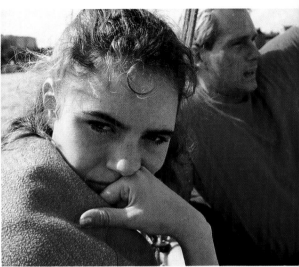

A telltale pain

A remarkable sight: the interior of the Fallopian tube.
Its finger-like projections—fimbriae—have captured
the ovum cell, which is still surrounded by thousands
of nutrient cells. *Below*, we see part of the ovum above
the forest of cilia that propel it forward.

Slight bleeding often accompanies ovulation, and if
the blood is shed against the peritoneum (the membrane surrounding the abdominal cavity) there may
be discomfort—*mittelschmerz*, as it is called. This
makes it easier for the woman to calculate the most
propitious time for conception.

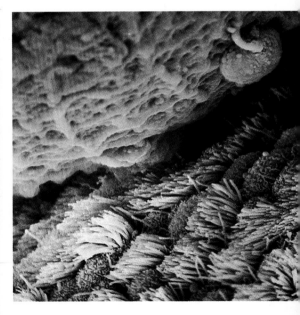

Ripening of the ovum

Once inside the Fallopian tube, the ovum is contained in an environment that suits it just as well as when it was inside the follicle. It now ripens increasingly, preparing itself for the encounter with the sperm. Rather than remaining immobile, it rolls slowly over the surface of the membrane folds while awaiting its male counterpart.

Meanwhile, the emptied follicle is being transformed. The hormone-producing cells that did not escape from the follicle during ovulation start growing and change their hormone production. Until now, the predominant hormone formed in the follicle was estrogen; this production now declines sharply and

Now the ovum is sailing through the narrow Fallopian tube, which is some 15 cm (about 6 inches) long. Beneath the ovum we see the cilia, which gently propel it forward. The liquid in the Fallopian tube washes away the nutrient cells surrounding the ovum. Here they still cluster about like a radiant wreath (*corona radiata*). Soon the ovum will be ready for fertilization and prepared to encounter the advances of the sperm. The chances of conceiving are at their highest in the next few hours.

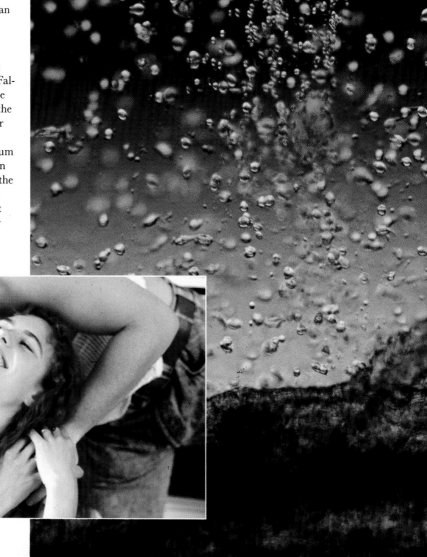

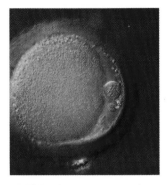

Half the chromosomes in the ovum, expelled when it ripens, collect in a cell called a polar body inside the ovum wall.

the corpus luteum starts producing progesterone instead.

A change in the information sent to the ovary by the brain and pituitary gland can result in more than one ovum being released at the time of ovulation: either one ovum from each of the ovaries or two (or more) from the same ovary. Twins or triplets may then be conceived. If this happens, the result is always non-identical (fraternal or dizygotic) twins, which may even be of different sexes. They are no more alike than any other two siblings. Identical (or monozygotic) twins, on the other hand, result from the fertilization of a single egg cell that then divides into two equal parts; thus, the fetuses are of the same sex and genetically identical.

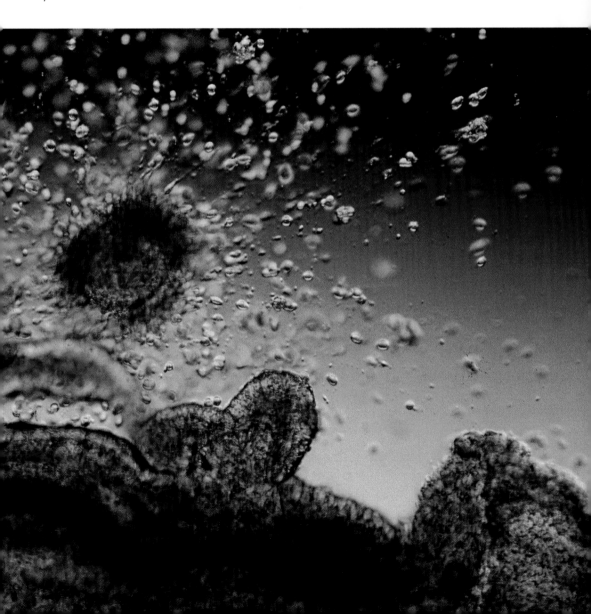

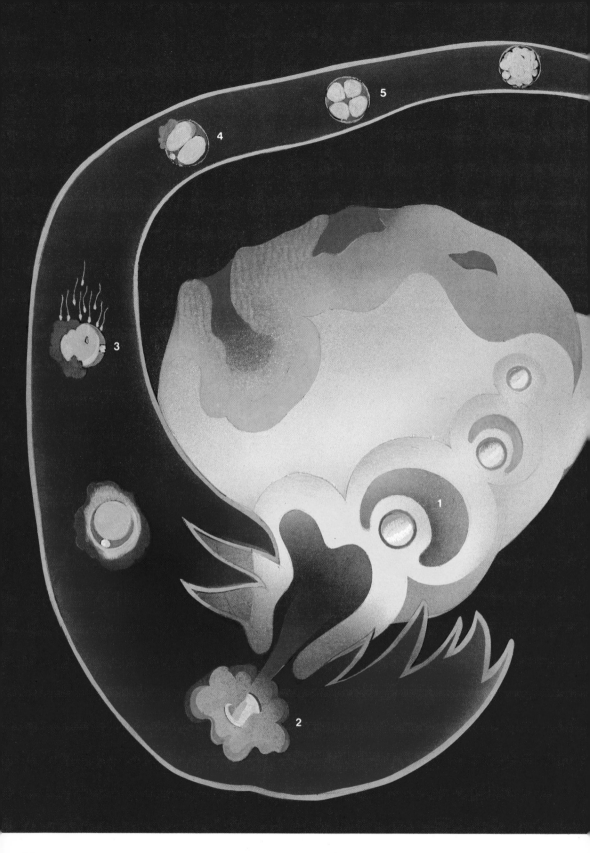

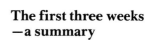

The first three weeks —a summary

(1) The follicles of the ovary grow, seek the ovary's surface and rupture. (2) The opening of the Fallopian tube sucks in the ovum, and the final ripening of the ovum takes place in the Fallopian tube while awaiting the sperm. (3) Fertilization takes place in the wide outer part of the tube. (4) Roughly 24 hours after the fusion, the first cell division takes place. (5) For some three or four days, the fertilized ovum remains in the Fallopian tube, dividing again and again. (6) The narrowest portion of the tube then opens and the fertilized ovum passes rapidly through the constricted passage into the uterus. (7) The fertilized ovum sheds its outer wall in order to be able to develop further. (8) The blastocyst can now expand freely, and seeks contact with the endometrium. (9) A few days later, the blastocyst is firmly attached to the endometrium. (10) Three weeks after fertilization, the blastocyst has become an embryo, and the first nerve cells have already formed.

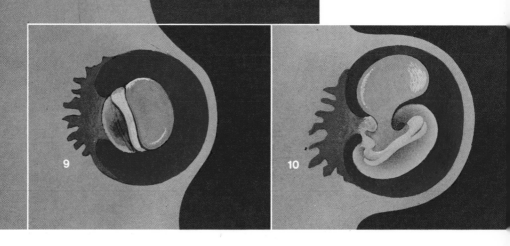

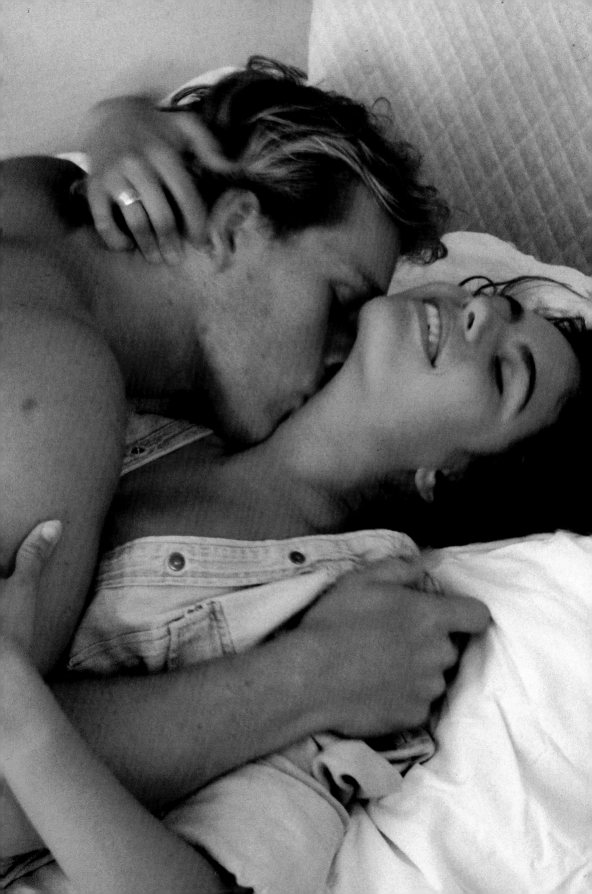

Fertilization

Fertilization, the moment the sperm and egg fuse and a new individual begins to form, has been until recently shrouded in mystery. It was known to take place in the Fallopian tube, deep inside the woman's body, but neither eye nor camera had penetrated these recesses. While our knowledge of this astonishing event is still incomplete, here, in pictures, we shall tell the story of how life begins.

Once drawn into the funnel of the Fallopian tube, the ovum comes to rest in the outer, broad portion of the tube. Surrounded by a sticky sheath of nutrient cells, the tiny ovum cell can barely be discerned. Sperm may already be in the Fallopian tube, or they may arrive later. The ovum, however, is capable of being fertilized for only some 24 hours. If no sperm arrive, it gradually degenerates and travels down through the Fallopian tube and uterus into the vagina. The woman then has her menstrual period two weeks later.

Many women feel increased sexual desire at the time of ovulation. This may be related to animals' estrous or mating periods, which in many species are tied in with the number of hours of light and darkness. Seasonal variations in childbearing appear to show that our sexual behavior still responds somewhat to changes in light.

Within a private, timeless world, events are taking place that will enrich and change forever the lives of two loving human beings.

In the picture to the *right*, sperm are attempting to move toward the womb through a barrier of cervical mucus. When ovulation takes place, channels of a hair's width form in the mucus, permitting the passage of sperm.

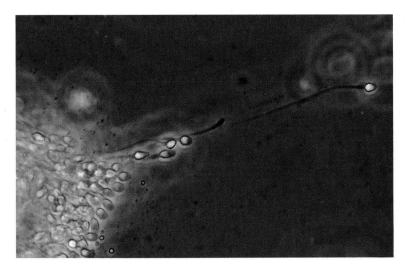

Five hundred million sperm at the start

During intercourse, sperm are ejaculated against the opening of the cervix at the far end of the vagina. Conditions in the vagina activate the sperm for about half an hour before they start moving up toward the uterus. The journey of 15–18 cm (about 6 to 7 inches) from vagina to Fallopian tube generally takes several hours. Some sperm are high-speed swimmers that, in favorable conditions, can reach the Fallopian tube in half an hour. Other sperm take numerous rests on the way, adhering in folds and recesses, but coming unstuck and struggling on. Their journey takes many hours, even days. During the journey, the sperm themselves change. They are affected by substances in the cervix, uterus and Fallopian tubes, becoming what is termed "capacitated," i.e. capable of fertilizing the ovum.

If there is no ovum in the Fallopian tube, the sperm swim

As though at the starting gate of a marathon, 500 million sperm set off toward an elusive finishing line: an ovum concealed in the Fallopian tube. Of this teeming crowd, only one can enter the ovum. For odds of 500 million to 1, a life-giving prize.

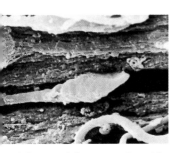

The initial danger — the acidity of the vagina — has been withstood. Now the sperm must make their way through one of the narrow passages in the cervical mucus. Only the fittest succeed.

back and forth in the broad portion of the tube, waiting, sometimes for several days. Some sperm emerge through the funnel and swim around in the abdominal cavity among the intestines and other organs. When ovulation occurs and the ovum enters the Fallopian tube, it exerts no particular force of chemical attraction on the sperm. Under a microscope, one can see how sperm quite simply swim past the ovum, at a distance of only a millimeter or so, going straight on until they encounter an obstacle.

The long survival time of the sperm, especially in the recesses of the cervix, means that intercourse four or five days before ovulation can result in fertilization. But conception is more likely if intercourse coincides with ovulation. The mucus of the cervix and uterus is then runny and transparent, permitting the sperm to swim upward to the ovum with ease.

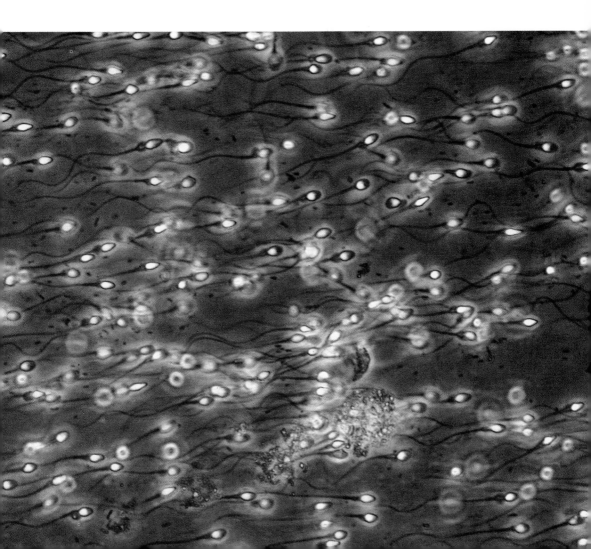

Obstacles on the way

Not only is the cervix filled with a usually impassable plug of mucus; it is also lined with recesses and dead ends in which many sperm adhere. Some are weak and tire rapidly. Most contenders get no farther than this first lap. *Right*, four who are still in the race.

The few million who continue soon encounter other problems. One is the white blood corpuscles—heavy artillery in the woman's immune system. Especially if she is suffering from a mild infection, they abound on the membrane surface. White blood cells kill everything that is foreign to the woman's own body, including sperm. In the picture, the white blood cells—macrophages and granulocytes—are pale yellow.

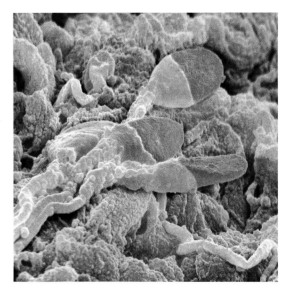

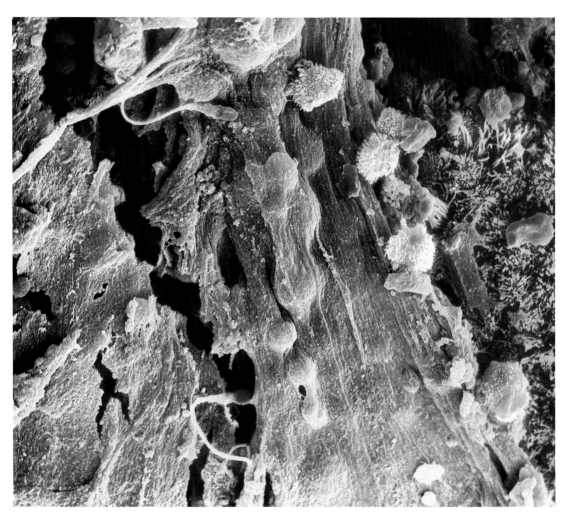

The energy pack

Immediately behind the head of the sperm lies a stack of mitochondria—the sperm's energy. This energy propels the sperm forward for many hours without refueling. Fertilization of the ovum usually takes place within less than 24 hours. When necessary the sperm can absorb more fuel from secretions in the Fallopian tube. Roughly a thousand tail-strokes drive the sperm forward one centimeter (less than half an inch), and each 10 centimeters (4 inches) of progress takes just over half an hour if no obstacles are encountered.

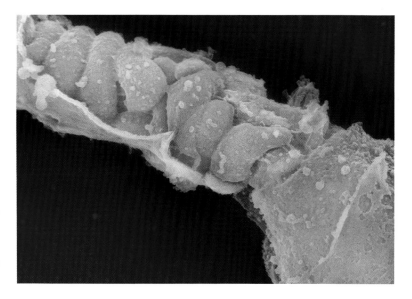

Forest of cilia

The sperm, *right*, is inside a thicket of cilia, tiny hairlike structures that line the walls of the cervix, uterus and Fallopian tubes. Between the clumps of reedlike cilia, glands are located. These produce a secretion that helps mature the sperm. The sperm constantly push their way forward, against the current created by the cilia beating toward the uterus.

The head of a sperm contains little more than the genetic material from the man: 23 chromosomes, with half the genes that the baby will possess, including the X or Y chromosome that determines the baby's sex.

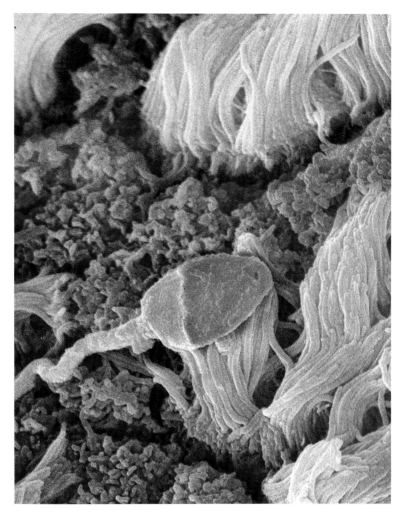

Two hours

First encounter

Like a planet in the solar system, suspended in space, the ovum cell is surrounded by the corona radiata—the luminous halo of nutrient cells. Notice how large it is compared with the tiny (red) sperm eagerly clustered against it in the upper right-hand part of the picture. This is the first encounter between the ovum and the hundred or so sperm that have succeeded in breaking through all the barriers. A mere hundred survivors out of an original 500 million!

Now they are drilling their heads through the ovum wall, beating with their tails—and causing the ovum to rotate slowly counterclockwise.

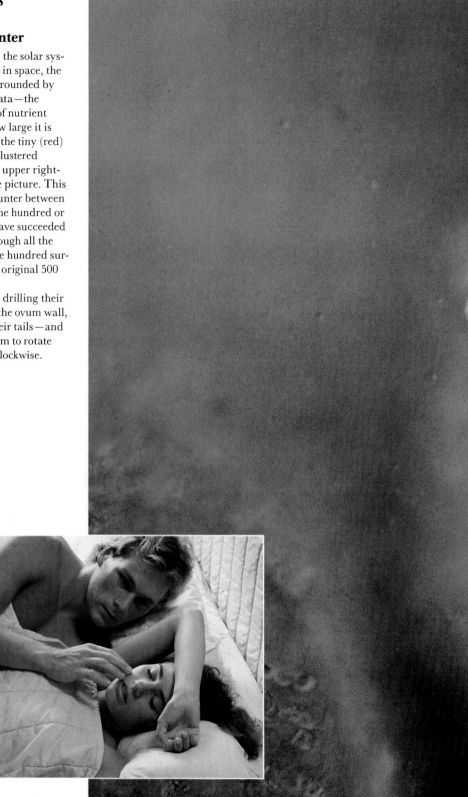

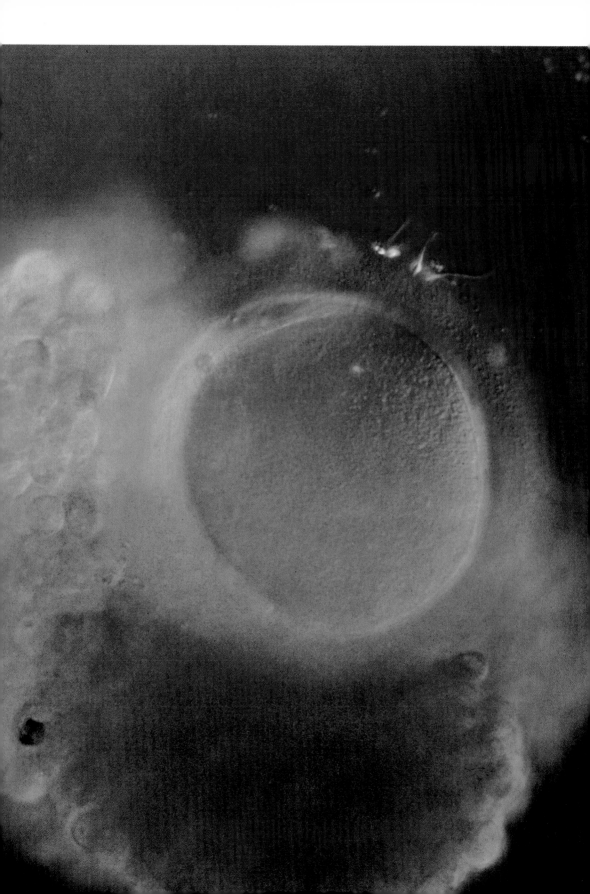

Stripping the ovum

When the sperm reach the ovum, it is still covered by the sheath of nutrient cells (*insert*). Some of these cells have performed their function and have been discarded during the passage through the Fallopian tube, but too many still remain for the sperm to penetrate the ovum. They must be cleared away (*large picture*). The cap of the sperm, the *acrosome*, gradually disappears and enzymes are released. These help the sperm to disrobe the egg. The pictures *below* show the infiltrating action of the sperm, two different degrees of magnification.

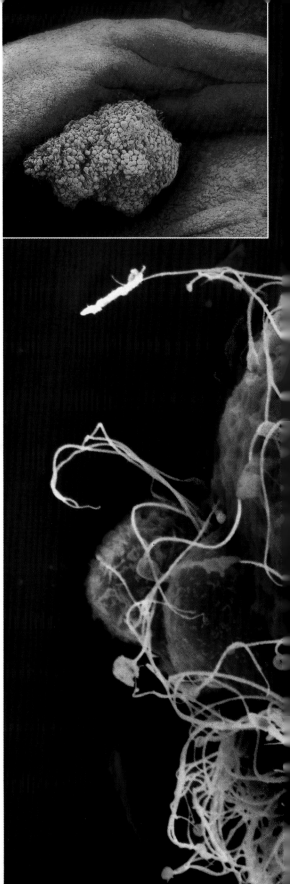

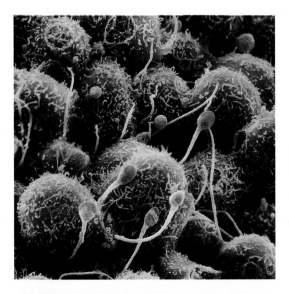

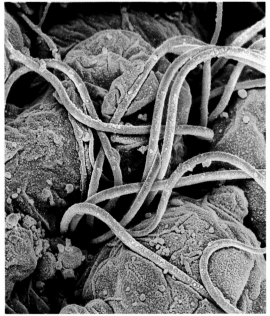

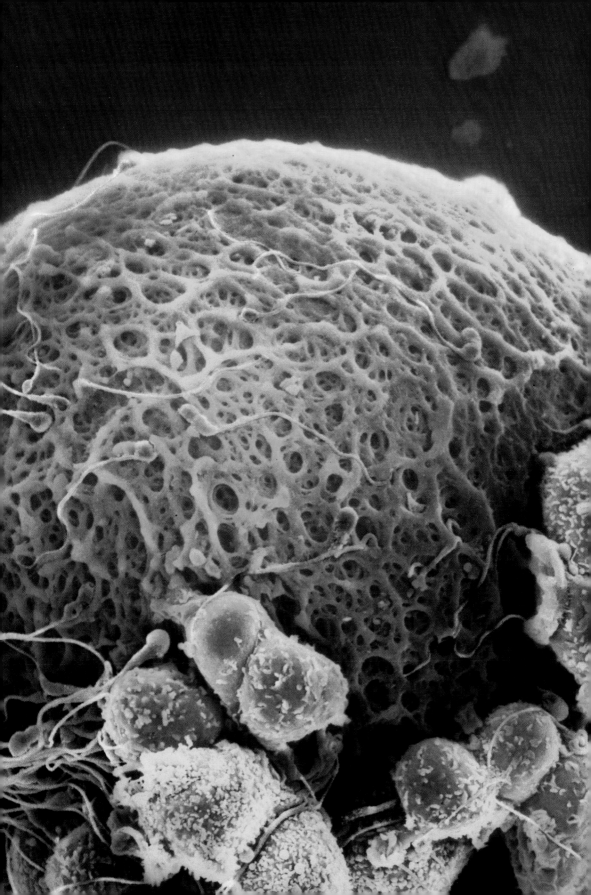

Fusion

Now a couple of hundred sperm have reached their destination, the ovum surrounded by a porous sheath of nutrient cells. Like a well-coordinated team, they penetrate one cell layer after another. In this cooperative venture, many sperm perish; others, which never attain full fertilization capacity, still join in the teamwork. After a few hours, at least some of the outer layers have been removed and the surface of the ovum is becoming exposed. Like a bird's egg, the human ovum has a kind of shell but one that is tough and elastic. This obstacle, too, can be overcome by vigorous sperm.

At the moment when a small number of sperm are on their way through the ovum wall, suddenly a single one breaks all the way through, penetrating the inner cell plasma of the ovum. Just then, something remarkable happens. The chemical composition of the ovum wall quickly changes, shutting out other sperm even if they have almost pierced it. This makes it impossible for additional sperm to fertilize the ovum. If this should happen, further development would sooner or later be arrested.

The excluded sperm continue to jostle around the ovum with undiminished strength and mobility for several days. Perhaps they serve no purpose; but they may help to promote the distinctive chemical environment that is so important to the ovum during its passage through the Fallopian tube.

As it struggles up toward the ovum (*below left*), each sperm wears a small "cap" termed an *acrosome*. Inside this cap are the proteins called enzymes that help the sperm break down the nutrient cells surrounding the ovum. While wearing the cap, no sperm can enter the ovum. *Below*, we see how the cap gradually dissolves.

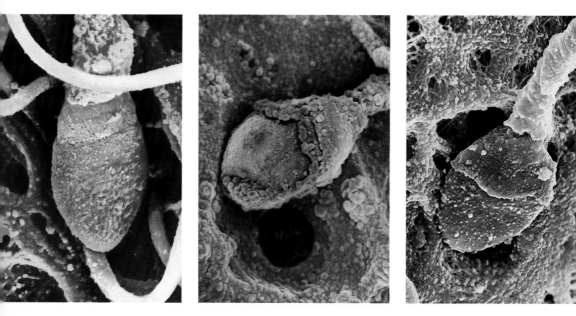

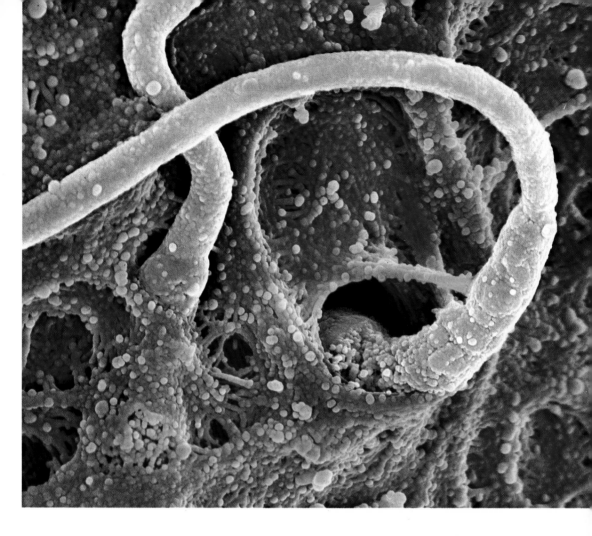

Several sperm may be on their way through the numerous small craters of the ovum wall. *Above*, the head of one sperm is visible, but only the tail of another. The leading sperm may now have only minutes to go before reaching the finishing line.

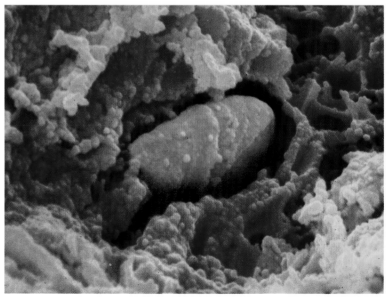

Right, we see the head of the winning sperm, visible inside the ovum. Now something remarkable occurs: the ovum shuts and bolts all the doors, preventing all other sperm from entering.

The winning sperm

This may well be the winner—the sperm that has now, finally, after at least 20,000 tail lashings, reached the ovum and penetrated its outer wall. It still has some way to go until it reaches the inner sanctum—the interior of the ovum cell. The head of the sperm has entered, and we see its tail and the middle section with its energy pack. The sperm works like a revolving drill, with its head rotated by the tail movements. *Insert*, the sperm head has now passed entirely through the ovum wall, and is about to penetrate the inner cell membrane.

The swimming sperm, the dancing ovum, all the secret phenomena inside the woman's body are matters of which the two expectant parents— the man and woman who love each other—are oblivious.

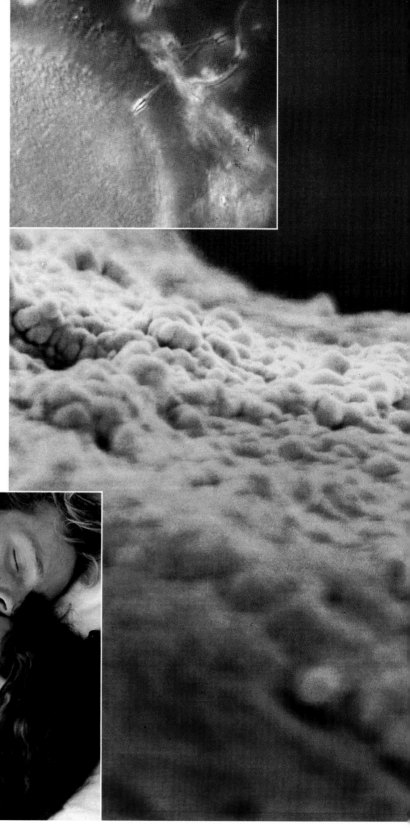

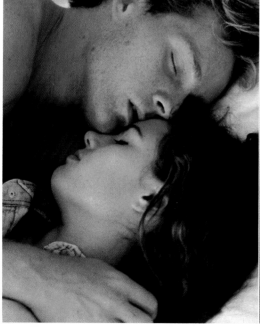

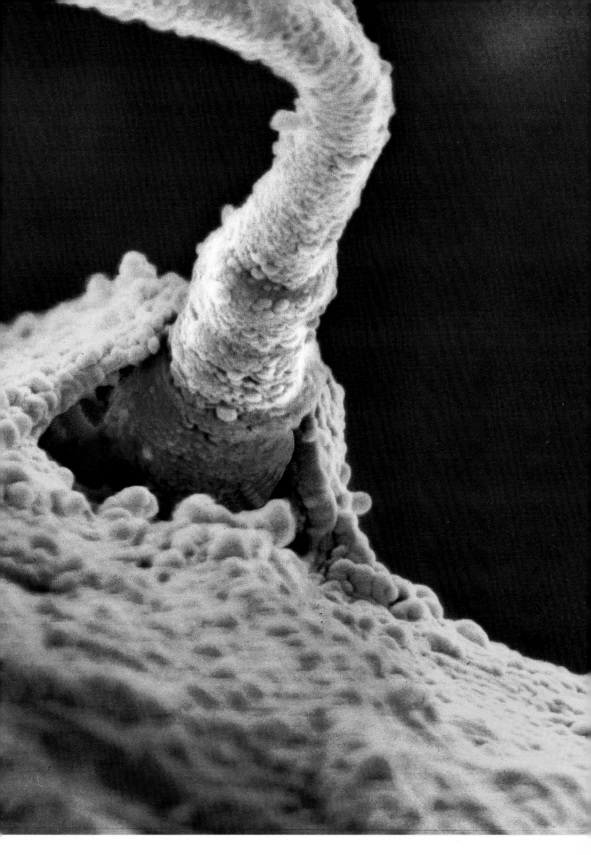

The sperm drops its tail

At the finish, as many as ten sperm simultaneously attempt to penetrate the ovum wall. As soon as one succeeds, a chemical signal goes from the ovum's inner membrane to the wall, which becomes impenetrable to other sperm. Even those that are halfway in are shut out. More than one set of chromosomes would be a disaster for the ovum.

Once the sperm has penetrated the ovum shell, its energetic tail has served its purpose and separates from the head (*below*).

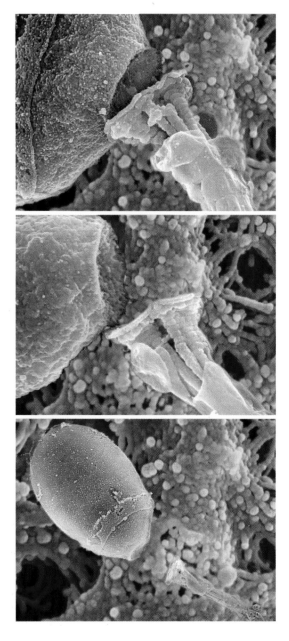

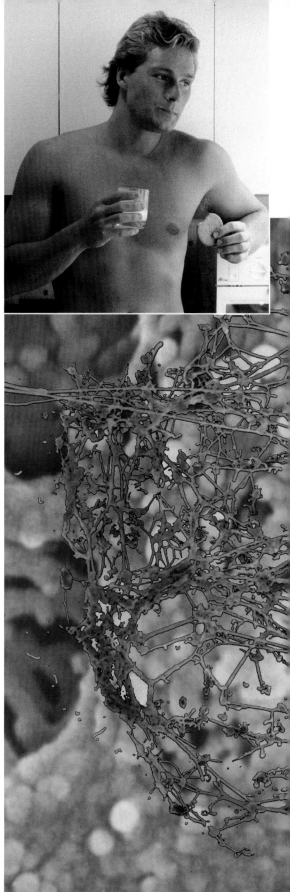

The sperm—a package of genes

In the large picture, we see the contents of the head of a sperm, six-hundredths of a millimeter long. The formerly tightly packed genes are spread out. The pattern looks chaotic, but there is in fact complete order. The molecules consist of DNA and proteins forming a rope-ladder pattern (*insert*).

The sperm's DNA spiral is the man's contribution to the hereditary blueprint of the baby-to-be. It contains the X chromosome that determines the baby will be female, or the Y chromosome that will make it a boy. Other characteristics stored in coded form are height, color of skin, eyes and hair—and the other characteristics of the hair, straightness or curliness—distinctive facial features, and so on.

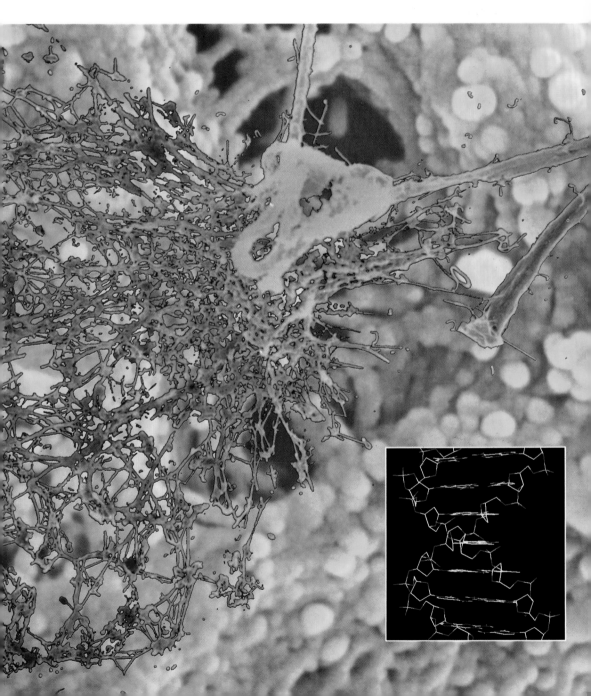

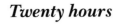

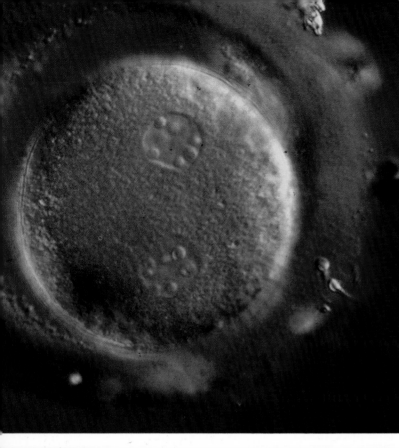

Twenty hours

The moment of fusion is at hand. The head of the sperm, with its genetic material, has penetrated the ovum's cell plasma and is steadily approaching the woman's genetic material, which is stored in a nucleus deep inside the ovum. Both nuclei are drawn inexorably toward each other, and soon fuse. Instantaneously, numerous hereditary characteristics of the new individual are determined.

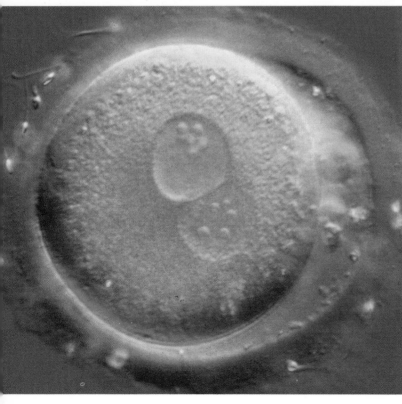

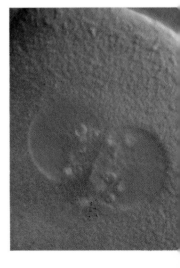

A new life begins

The head of the victorious sperm, with its genetic blueprint, now lies inside a tiny nucleus in the ovum. The ovum's genetic material, too, has been concentrated in a tiny nucleus. Inside these nuclei, there are round structures in which copying of the DNA message takes place. Some repairs of genes damaged in transport are also carried out. The inner substance of the cell moves vigorously, as if to force together the genetic material that is to make up the new individual. At first, the nuclei are located far apart, with the head of the sperm on the periphery and the ovum nucleus in the center, but they slowly approach each other and fuse. The outer walls of the nuclei then dissolve, and everything is swallowed up by the cell plasma of the ovum.

Roughly 12 hours after the fusion of the chromosomes, the first cell division takes place, and divisions then continue at intervals of 12 to 15 hours.

Long after fertilization, sperm with lashing tails may be seen trying in vain to enter the interior of the ovum. They may keep this up for several days. Seen under a microscope, during *in vitro* fertilization, there are sometimes a hundred or more sperm on the ovum's surface, and one can see how the tail movements make the ovum rotate counterclockwise. It is conceivable that excluded sperm may play a significant part in causing the ovum to start rolling along the mucous membrane surface of the Fallopian tube on its way to the uterus.

At this stage, no chemical substances or other mechanisms are yet signaling to the woman about developments deep inside her body.

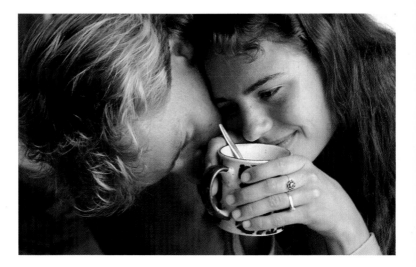

Unaware of events in the depths of her body, the young woman and her partner rejoice in their love.

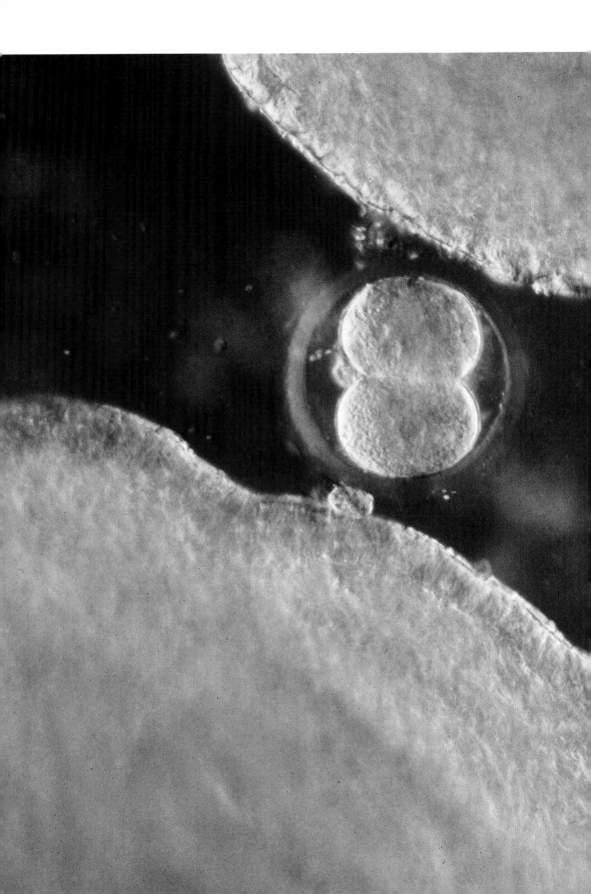

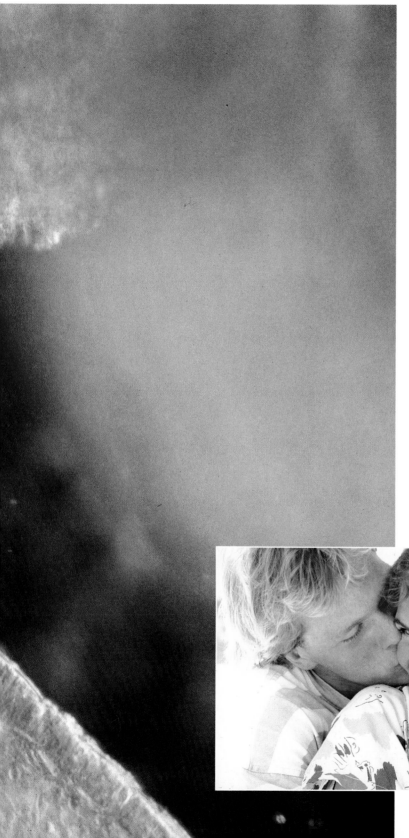

First portrait

A few hours after the nuclei have fused, the fertilized ovum divides for the first time, with a powerful force. It now has two cells, each containing genes from both the mother and the father. Moving slowly toward the uterus, propelled forward by millions of cilia in the Fallopian tube, the cells divide anew every 12 to 15 hours. The Fallopian tube harbors risks for the growing cells: they may, for example, adhere in one of the many folds of the mucous membrane. If they continue to grow there, the result is a tubal, or ectopic, pregnancy.

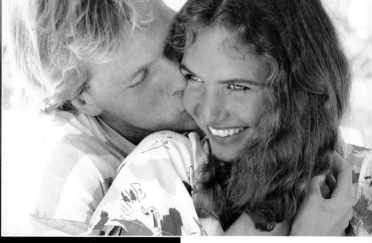

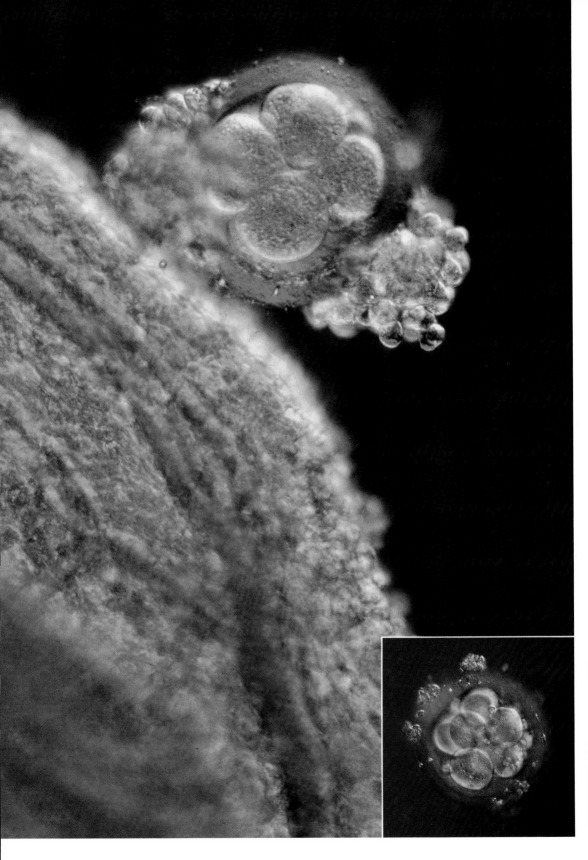

Two days

The divisions continue: four visible cells and perhaps eight all together are on their way through the Fallopian tube's thicket of cilia to the uterus. The clump of cells is embedded in nutrient cells that nourish it. In the *insert*, it has developed into 16 cells. The following picture shows the morula stage (*morula* = mulberry), and *far right* we see the blastocyst, now comprising about a hundred cells. Here, it is passing through the narrowest portion of the Fallopian tube just before entering the uterus. It is a tight squeeze, and the blastocyst must push its way forward between the folds.

The long journey

The ovum remains in the Fallopian tube for about three days after fertilization, dividing repeatedly during its slow journey down toward the uterus. The fertilized ovum normally has no direct contact with the mucous membrane of the Fallopian tube, but substances flow through the membrane toward the tiny clump of cells that create a favorable habitat. On the actual surface of the mucous membrane millions of tiny cilia keep beating in the same direction—toward the uterus. The muscles of the Fallopian tube also contract periodically and give the ovum a gentle push.

In the transition between the wider and narrower parts of the Fallopian tube there is a barrier in the form of a sphincter muscle which is impassable to the fertilized ovum despite its small size. However, this muscle now suddenly relaxes and the passage leading to the uterus opens. We have learned that the sphincter's relaxation is primarily due to the secretion of progesterone—now beginning to be produced copiously by the corpus luteum, formed from what was previously the ovarian follicle.

The passage through this narrow part of the Fallopian tube usually takes a few hours; the fertilized ovum must force and jostle its way through the mucous membrane folds, without getting stuck.

Once inside the uterus, one of the most critical phases of early development is over. Now the fertilized ovum, which has become what is known as a blastocyst, faces new tasks: to attach itself to the uterine lining and to signal its presence to the mother. There is plenty of room in the uterus. Soon the blastocyst will "hatch" and rupture its transparent wall.

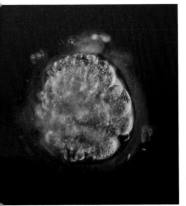

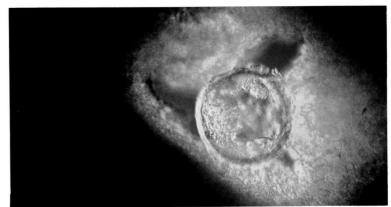

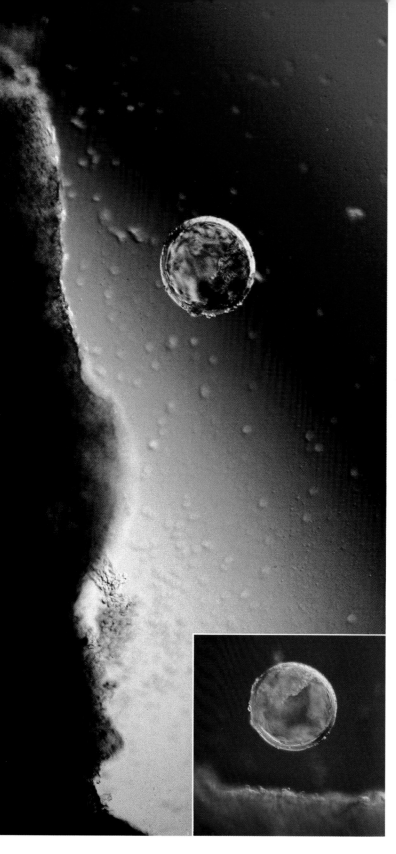

Four days

Surrounded by its transparent wall, the zona pellucida, the blastocyst now glides into the uterus. Its journey is still not over: now it must settle down in the endometrium. The series of pictures *below* show this "lunar landing." The blastocyst is feeling its way over the mucous membrane of the uterus, but cannot yet become implanted because of its shell-like sheath. The last picture in the series shows the blastocyst breaking out of the sheath and setting itself free. Only now can the cell mass expand before it attaches itself to the welcoming, soft and thickened membrane. Notice that the egg is now larger than the discarded sheath.

At this stage, the cells in the blastocyst also begin to differentiate, as the large picture, *right*, shows. The upper, light half is the rudimentary embryo, while the future placenta can be seen below.

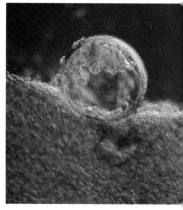

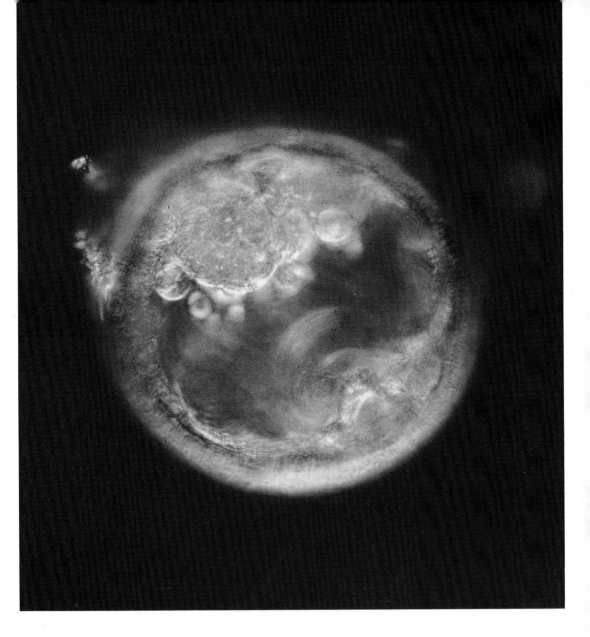

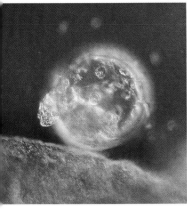

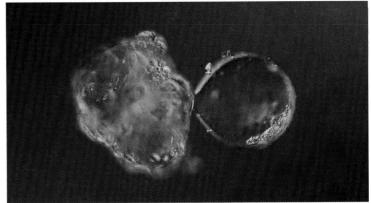

Implantation

Eight days

The uterine lining, the endometrium, has been prepared by hormones from the ovary to receive the fertilized ovum. However, the blastocyst often takes several days to select a suitable site for attachment and implantation. It usually becomes embedded near the "ceiling" of the uterus.

When the blastocyst has finally come to rest and established contact with the endometrium, an intensive chemical exchange of information between it and the mother's body begins. Proteins, such as hormones, formed in the blastocyst enter the woman's bloodstream. These can be detected by means of a blood test; in this way, pregnancy can be verified with a high degree of certainty well before the first menstrual period has been missed.

Several of the substances formed in the blastocyst during implantation influence the woman's immune system, at least locally to start with. Since the ovum, once fertilized, consists largely of "foreign" proteins, the woman's body should in fact reject the intruder. But, thanks to certain cells in the blastocyst, which produce chemical substances that weaken the woman's immune system in the uterus, the blastocyst is not rejected and finds a nurturing home.

We have discovered in recent years that some women who miscarry repeatedly suffer from a defect in this part of the immune system, and that their miscarriages can be prevented if this defect is repaired. The more we learn about these amazing mechanisms, the more astounding human conception and all the precisely designed functions of the human body appear.

Women who are sensitive to hormonal changes may already have an inkling as to what is going on.

The blastocyst has landed! Like a raspberry on a cake, it sinks slightly into its foundation. The clump is now made up of several hundred cells. Implantation is facilitated by the formation of small protuberances of sugar molecules on the blastocyst's surface (*below left*). This "landing apparatus" corresponds to similar molecules in the endometrium. A really secure foothold is required. Hormones also help the blastocyst settle in. Progesterone (shown in crystalline form *below*) is secreted by the ovary. Its task is to signal to the pituitary gland in the brain that the woman is pregnant and no menstrual period should take place.

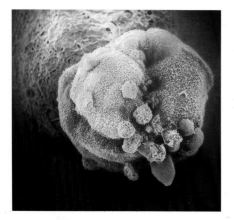

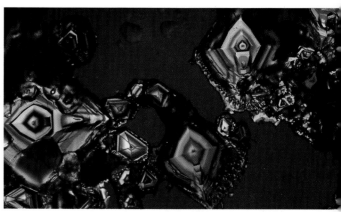

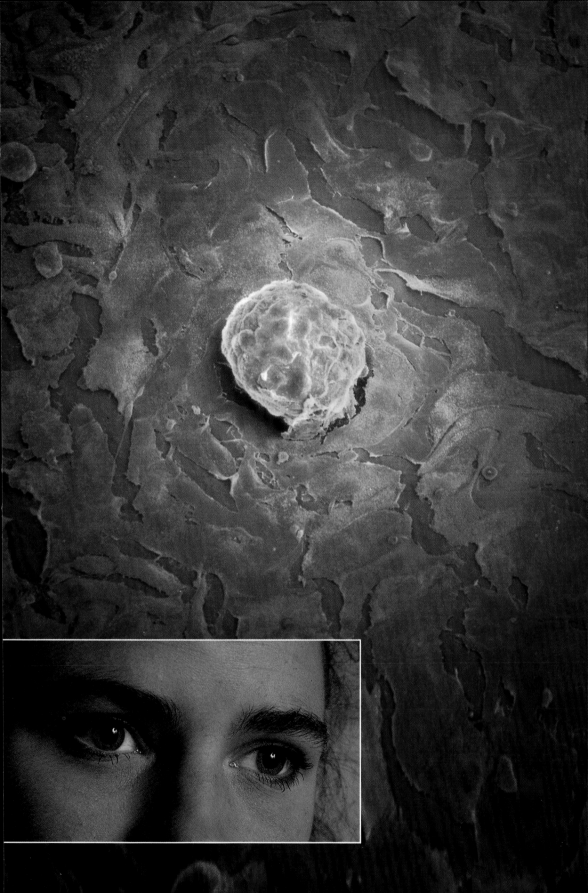

Eight days old

At first, just the actual landing site in the uterus is affected by signals from the blastocyst. Then the endometrium is transformed throughout the uterus, becoming thicker. The passage down to the cervix is sealed by a plug of mucus, and the muscles of the uterine wall become softer and more elastic. All these rapid changes create a favorable and sheltered environment for the growing embryo. Beneath the endometrium, blood vessels start to move toward the surface to facilitate the exchange of nutrients. Each of the hormonal changes in the woman's body triggered off by the blastocyst's signals must be complete and take place in the correct chronological order; otherwise, the outer layers of the endometrium are shed as during an ordinary menstrual period, producing a very early miscarriage.

A careful examination of the blastocyst's surface reveals that almost every cell is unlike every other. Some have long projections, others have short ones and some lack projections altogether. This is called cell differentiation. Until about the eight-cell stage, all the cells look the same and serve exactly the same purpose. How, then, do cells know what to become and which organ of the body to form? This is one of the major secrets of life that still eludes us, an intense field of scientific investigation.

A vital event: eight days after fertilization, the blastocyst (now comprising some 200 cells) secretes a mucus that proclaims its presence in the uterus. The new, developing individual has a different genetic makeup from that of the mother in whose body it lives. If the mother's immune system were to detect the alien tissue, it might reject it—just as when organs are transplanted between people. By chemical means, however, the mucus from the blastocyst creates a sanctuary for the embryo in the uterus through what might be called a non-aggression pact at the cellular level.

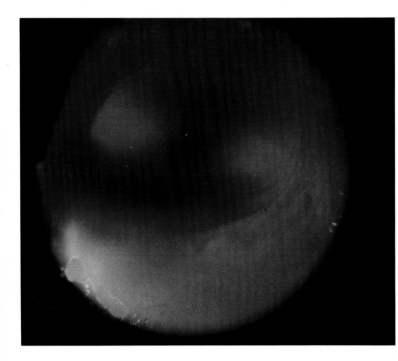

Our first home

Interior of the upper portion of the uterus, where the Fallopian tubes (the lighter patches above) are visible. Most blastocysts implant here. The uterus expands enormously during pregnancy. The drawing shows the usual location of implantation in the uterus.

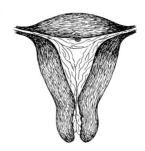

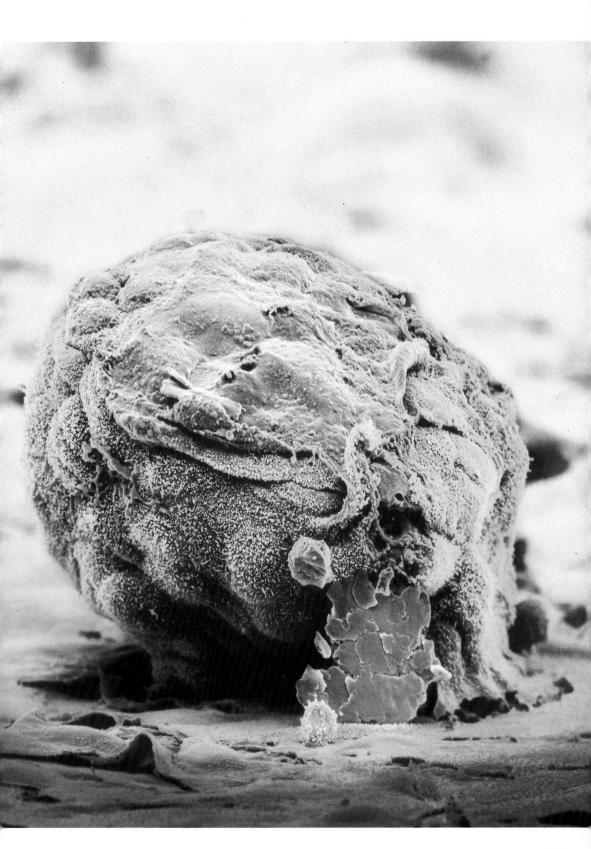

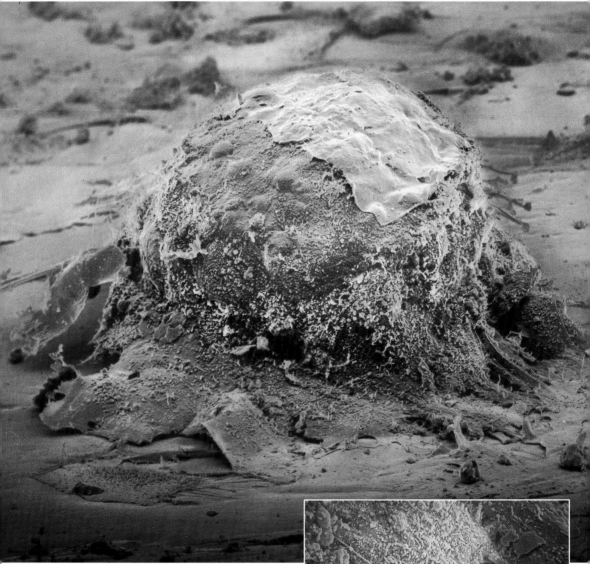

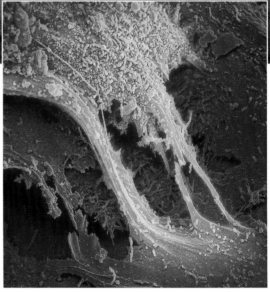

Eleven days

The blastocyst swells, the cells divide roughly twice a day and now—on the 12th day—they number a couple of thousand. The blastocyst is securely anchored in the endometrium; here and there, veritable cables are visible (*insert*). Protuberances like this probably develop into the amniotic sac, the umbilical cord and the placenta. In due course nourishment and waste products will be exchanged in a highly organized fashion. It is hard to imagine how this cluster of cells can come to resemble its parents in less than nine months.

Dangers on the way

Early *miscarriages*—so early that women are not even aware that they are pregnant—are very common. This usually means that chromosomes are damaged, or that there are too few or too many. The barrier built into the ovum wall to prevent more than one sperm from fertilizing serves to prevent such flaws in its further development. Ova fertilized by two or more sperm may grow to a relatively advanced stage but, since too much genetic material has entered the ovum, eventually development goes wrong. This is one cause of an early miscarriage. Another reason for miscarriage, one that is not especially unusual, is a sperm with some defect in its chromosomal composition. Thus, miscarriage is often nature's way of protecting itself against genetic deviations; and sperm are, in fact, more often the cause than the ovum.

Sometimes the fertilized ovum becomes stuck in the Fallopian tube and cannot proceed. This is often due to damage in the tube. It may be scarred from a previous infection or operation. If the woman is unlucky, the fertilized ovum attaches itself and starts to grow right there in the wall of the Fallopian tube. This is known as a tubal or *ectopic pregnancy*. At first, everything develops normally: the tiny embryo grows and increases in size, the woman experiences the normal signs of pregnancy and a test of her urine usually gives a positive result. Soon, however, the narrowness of the Fallopian tube means that the embryo runs out of space. Because it has tremendous growing power it will eventually cause the tube to rupture, causing a hemorrhage. An emergency operation is then necessary, to remove the embryo and often part of the Fallopian tube as well.

For partially unknown reasons, ectopic pregnancies have become more common in the Western world over the past 10 to 15 years. In urban areas, the rate has been rising; of approximately 70 pregnancies, one is ectopic. The growing number of pelvic infections is considered a major contributory factor, but not all cases of ectopic pregnancy can be explained plausibly. In developing countries, undetected and untreated ectopic pregnancies cause the deaths of many young women.

If the uterine cavity is damaged, or malformed, the ovum may become implanted in various unfavorable sites, resulting in problems later in pregnancy. If the placenta should expand to cover the cervical os, the inner opening to the cervix (this is termed *placenta praevia*), the baby's exit from the uterus is blocked. A delivery by cesarean section is then necessary.

Hormonal changes

Becoming pregnant is a dramatic change with a global effect on the woman—both body and soul. As early as a week or so after ovulation, i.e. well before she misses her first menstrual period, the woman often knows instinctively that something has happened inside her, and the pregnancy test is merely an almost obvious confirmation of something she already knew. The first signs are often swelling, tender breasts, slight nausea and heightened sensitivity to odors and flavors. Many women become extremely tired and find it difficult to concentrate on their work, although the only thing that has actually happened so far is that a clump of cells barely a millimeter (.04 inch) across has dug itself into the uterine wall and begun to signal its presence and its needs.

The tiny group of cells divides into two parts: one will form the embryo itself and the other the rudimentary placenta. The cells of the placenta almost immediately start forming a placental hormone called *human chorionic gonadotropin* (hCG for short). One of the first tasks of this hormone is to notify the ovaries that the woman is now pregnant and no more ovulations are needed for a long time. But the signal also directs the ovary to help retain the endometrium and prevent the menstrual period

Tired and irritable

As early as ten days after ovulation, a woman may begin to notice that something unusual is under way in her body. Her breasts become enlarged and tender, and she may tire easily and feel irritable. Her partner does not always understand what this is all about, and may perhaps think he has said or done something wrong.

The reason is to be found in the endometrium: a cluster of cells measuring barely a millimeter in diameter. They have set in train an upheaval in the woman's entire being. One of these changes is an increase in progesterone, which first comes from the ovary and is then produced by the placenta (*below*, in the form of crystals).

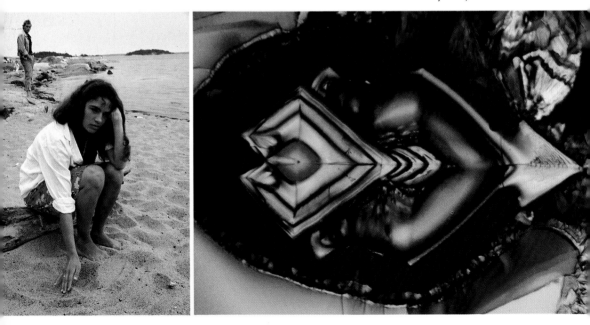

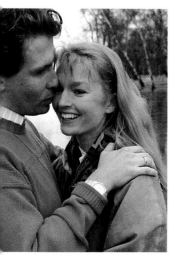

Couples who are eager to have a baby greet these changes in the woman's body with joyful expectation.

which would expel the embryo from the uterus. The ovary accomplishes this by forming more progesterone, which is transported to the uterus in the bloodstream. It is this hormone that causes the endometrium to grow and flourish.

The interplay between hCG and progesterone gives the woman all her signs of pregnancy. In fact a pregnancy test could be based on either of these hormones. Progesterone is present in small quantities whether the woman is pregnant or not, while the placental hormone, hCG, is present only in pregnancy. The most sensitive pregnancy tests are done with blood samples, but very soon a large quantity of hCG begins to be secreted in the urine, and a pregnancy test can be carried out on a urine sample. Nowadays, using simple and rapid urinary hCG tests, chemists can ascertain pregnancy as early as a week after ovulation, i.e. a week before the woman would normally have had her menstrual period.

Very early in pregnancy, the placenta itself starts to help the ovaries produce progesterone, this very important hormone required throughout pregnancy. As early as seven or eight weeks after the last menstrual period, the ovaries are in fact no longer needed. The placenta is now capable of producing all the hormones necessary to enable the fetus to develop normally.

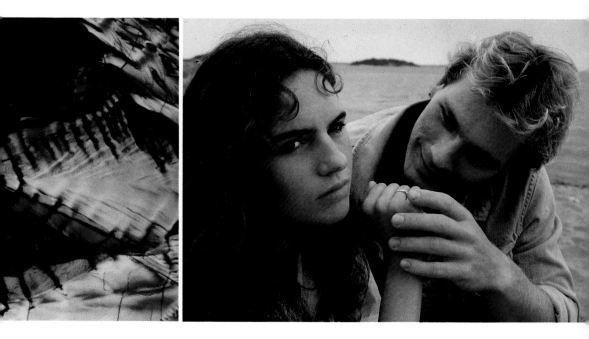

We're going to have a baby!

Now the woman is anxious for a definite answer: Am I pregnant or not? These days, this is a simple matter. Together, she and her partner simply walk down to the pharmacy and buy a pregnancy test. The test is based on the reaction in the urine between the pregnancy hormone hCG and a chemical added to it. The hormone is formed in the placenta and borne in the bloodstream to the ovaries, where it stimulates production of progesterone. Thus, hCG is part of the hormonal system that protects the embryo against the

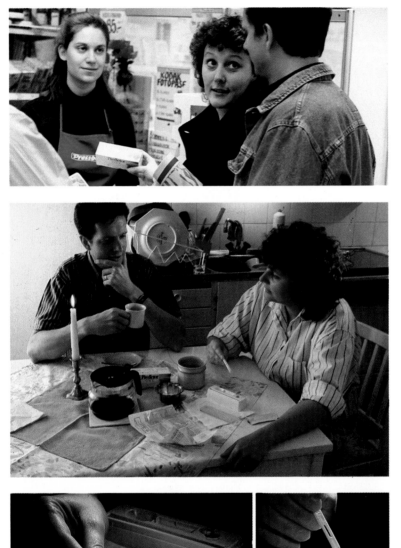

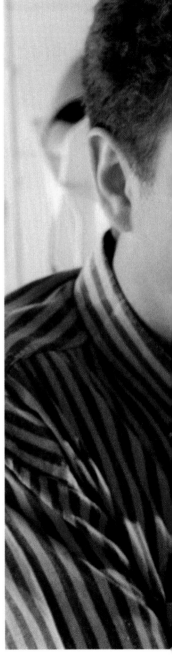

occurrence of a menstrual period. Bleeding would strip away the endometrium, including the embryo. The pregnancy test involves dipping a strip of paper in the woman's urine and observing the color. It's red—she's pregnant! The test is extremely sensitive: as early as a week or so after a missed menstrual period, a definite result can be obtained. Another way of finding out is to bring a small sample of early-morning urine to a clinic or doctor's office. Then the woman gets a quick answer. For many expectant mothers an immediate talk with a doctor, nurse or midwife is reassuring. So many questions arise.

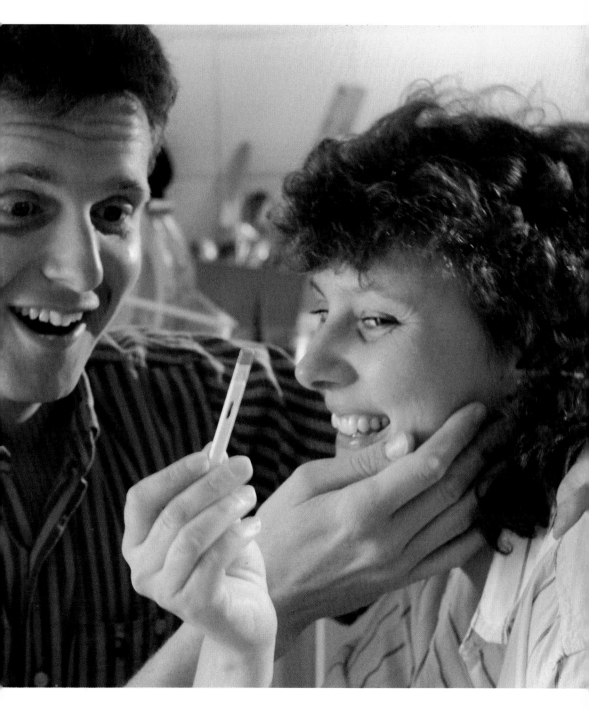

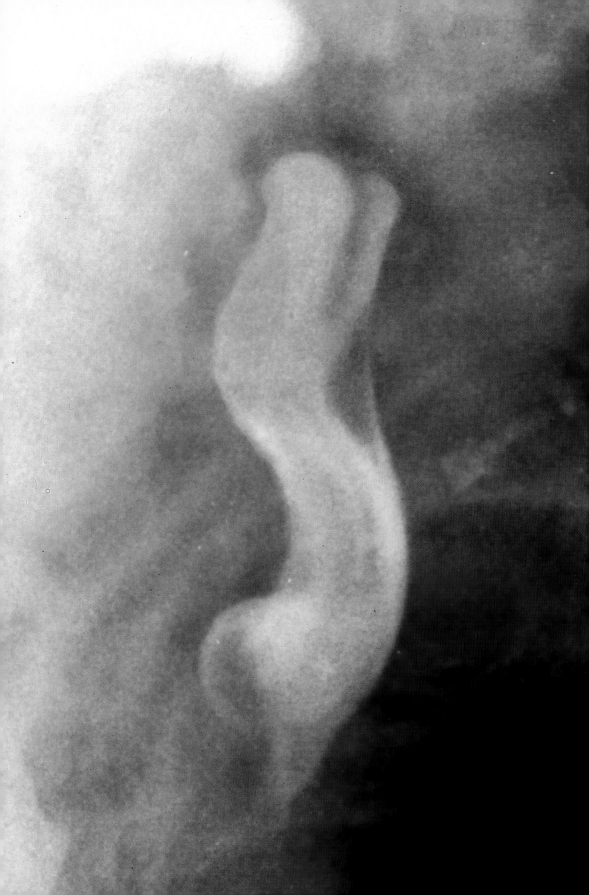

The First Few Weeks

Every day during the first few weeks after conception, new developments occur which are crucial to future growth. Fertilization, the safe journey through the Fallopian tube, implantation in the uterus, the first signals to the ovaries and the brain, early cell division and the emergence of a nurturing placenta: each event is as vital as the last. When one considers all the possible hazards and disturbances that could interrupt this process, the development and birth of a new human being seems all the more miraculous.

As early as three weeks after fertilization, parts of the future human body can already be identified. At this stage, one can clearly see how the outer layer—the embryo's skin—is thickening along the middle line of the body and forming two lengthwise folds. Between the folds is a groove that closes to form a tube known as the neural tube, which will soon develop into the spinal cord and brain. At one end of this tube, the rudimentary brain forms a swelling. Nerves from the brain stem and the primitive backbone are also beginning to develop. The tiny body may now be seen to have three different layers of cells, known as *germ layers* or *cell layers*. Out of these three layers, all the different organs of the body are gradually being formed. At this very early time, the rounded cluster of cells has already begun to assume a certain shape and characteristics recognizable as those of a mammal.

The embryo still does not look human. When the menstrual period is just over a week overdue, a head is barely perceptible surrounding the brain, with a large, gaping mouth opening. Immediately below the head, the embryonic heart is beginning to be formed and to beat. The lower part of the body still resembles a pointed tail. The cells are now beginning to specialize more and more.

This is an extremely sensitive period, the slightest defect in the elaborate program may lead to malformations that will affect the emerging individual throughout life. Fortunately, however, if the defects are excessive, nature has built-in safeguards: the embryo will cease to develop, and the woman will suffer an early miscarriage.

Who would believe that this amorphous creature, just under 2 mm (about .08 inch) long, has a good chance of being born as a little human being in eight months time? The parents, meanwhile, unaware of how things look inside the mother's abdomen, are content with the fact that the miracle has taken place: they are expecting a baby!

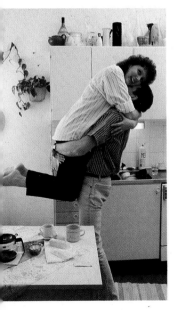

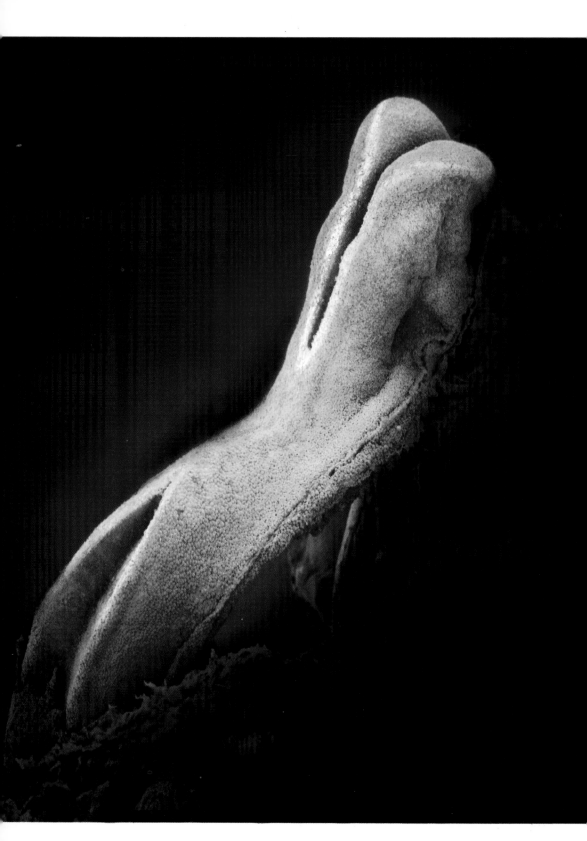

Three weeks

Three weeks after conception, the human embryo is barely 2 mm (.08 inch) long. The genes have just begun to concentrate development in the three germ (cell) layers from which all the body's organs are to emerge.

Left, we see how the outer layer, the embryo's skin, is cleft by the groove of the neural tube. The swelling above is the rudimentary forebrain. Below this may be glimpsed the rudimentary heart, branchial (gill) arches, which will later form the face and throat, and inner ear. The neural tube is open at the top and bottom but closed in the middle, where the trunk is.

Below, a detail of the embryo's head end, where the paler areas are the human being's first, primitive nerve cells; *below right*, the superficial nerve cells, greatly enlarged.

The heart starts beating

One of the great puzzles of biology is the question of how each cell knows what it is to become. After all, right from the start and throughout their existence, cells have the same code built into the cell nucleus. Yet different portions of this message are expressed in different cells—why and exactly how, no one yet knows.

From the *outer germ* (or *cell*) *layer*, the backbone, brain and nerves are formed. The primitive nerve cells that are clearly distinguishable three weeks after fertilization have only the suggestion of bulges projecting toward their nearest neighbors. The transmission of nerve impulses that may cause a body movement or register a sensation comes much later. The tiny embryo definitely lacks consciousness at this stage. The outer layer also gives rise to the skin, complete with hair and both sebaceous and sweat glands. The *middle layer* is destined for other organs: it forms the deeper layer of the skin (the dermis), the bones and the muscles. The middle layer also builds up blood and lymph vessels, produces blood cells and the heart muscle which in turn develop a primitive bloodstream. Ovaries, testicles and kidneys also develop from the middle layer. Meanwhile, the *inner layer* has simultaneously started to form a simple intestinal tube lined with mucous membranes, from which—remarkably enough—the lungs and urinary tract also develop. All the organs from the different cell layers must now become coordinated, so that the entire system can start to function. Every day during this period, the embryo "tries out" its newly combined systems to ensure that everything is functioning according to plan.

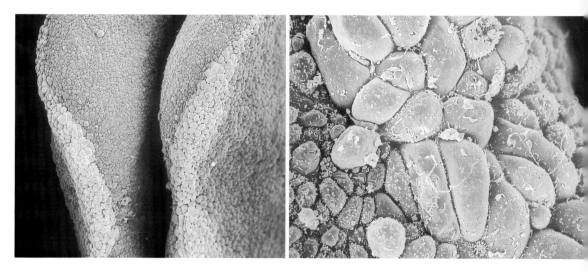

Neither fish nor fowl

Man is a vertebrate, and this is now increasingly visible. On each side of the neural groove, 40 small blocks of bone called *somites* are formed from the middle layer. Thirty-two, or sometimes 33, of these blocks become vertebrae, while the tail gradually regresses. From the 12 vertebrae at the level of the chest, known as the thoracic vertebrae, ribs start to grow around the rudimentary lungs. All the vertebrae are held together by elastic connective tissue and muscles which keep the backbone flexible. Between the vertebrae, bunches of nerves emerge which spread to form a network throughout the body.

Between the mouth opening and the heart, six projections grow outward from the cervical (neck) section of the vertebral column. At this stage they resemble fish gills. One of these projections becomes the lower jaw, while the others form the neck and face. The really human characteristics, and differences in facial features between individuals, will develop much later.

Day after day, the process of creation continues, with millions of cells forming custom-made building blocks. During this phase, the embryo is particularly sensitive to influences which could cross the placenta, such as drugs or certain infections.

Four weeks

The basic human design is beginning to emerge. The embryo pictured *right*, 4 weeks old and some 6 mm (about ¼ inch) long, shows the clear rudiments of brain and backbone. Its heart pumps blood to the liver and into the aorta. The bulge above the heart is the branchial arches. *Below left*, we see the embryo from the front, and *upper right* shows it from above. The two babies are photographed from the same angles.

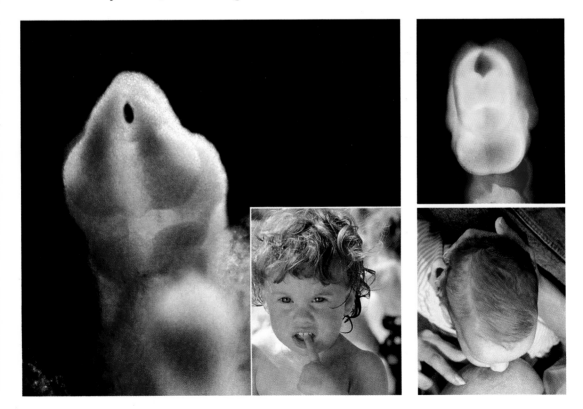

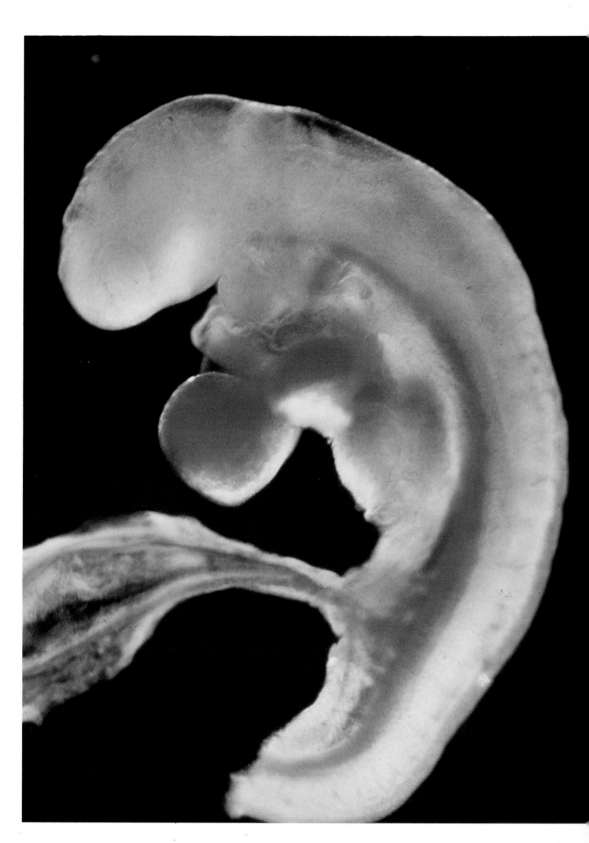

Tiny prehistoric creature

With its grotesquely large head and its tail—and with the clearly demarcated vertebrae—the 4½-week-old embryo resembles a prehistoric animal more than anything else. Beneath the rudimentary eye we see the branchial arches and the heart; arm and leg buds are also in evidence. Length: 6 mm (¼ inch).

Below: five days later, the embryo has almost doubled its length and is now growing a millimeter a day. Here we see it in its home environment, the amniotic sac, and suspended in its soft shock absorber, the amniotic fluid. The round ball under the head is the heart, and to the left are the backbone's developing vertebrae and the tail.

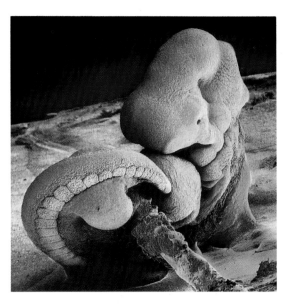

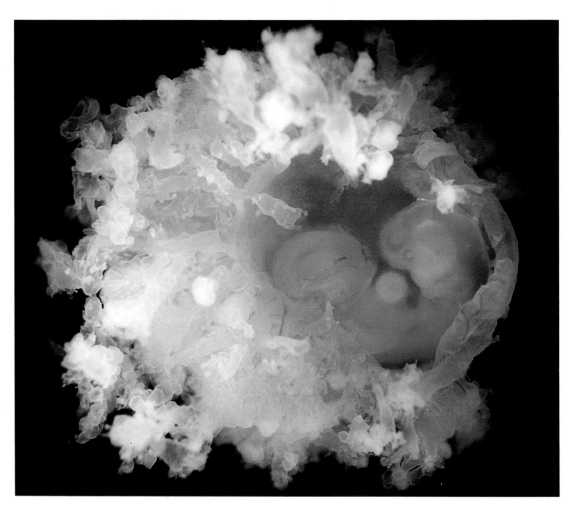

The placenta

The placenta rapidly works its way into the endometrium and its blood vessels. It may be likened to a busy freight terminal: here, nourishment is absorbed from the mother's blood and the embryo rids itself of waste products from its own metabolic system. Illustrated *right* are (1) the placenta with the umbilical cord, (2) the outer fetal membrane, the *chorion*, (3) the yolk sac, (4) the inner fetal membrane, the *amnion*, (5) the embryo's head end, with its rudimentary brain and eyes, (6) the fetal heart and (7) the beginning of a backbone.

Below, an embryo just over five weeks after conception, one centimeter (.4 inch) long. The heart and liver are strikingly large in relation to the body. The hands and feet are as yet merely small buds.

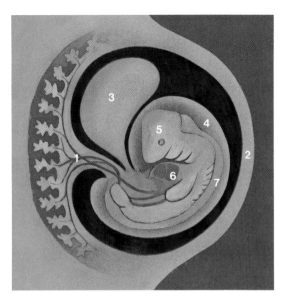

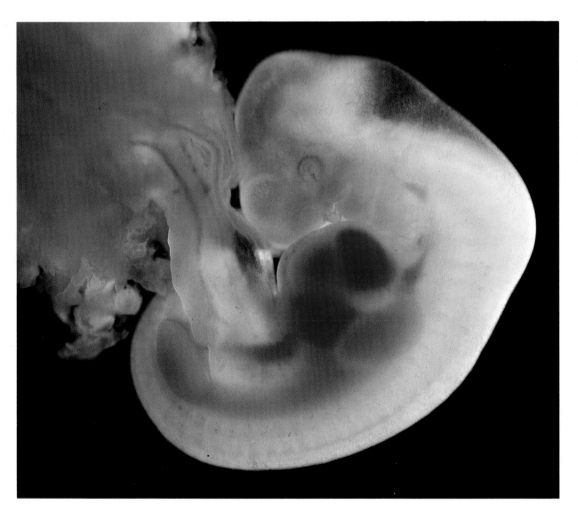

How do we know what stage an embryo has reached in its development? From numerous investigations of women who have suffered miscarriages, accurate measurements and calculations have been made. From this we know that the embryo is roughly one centimeter (.4 inch) long five weeks after fertilization. Nowadays, these measurements can be done more simply. Without in any way damaging the embryo, we can obtain information about the pregnancy by means of ultrasound as early as five weeks from the start of the last menstrual period. Initially, the ultrasound images show only a small membrane sac with the tiny bright spot of an embryo that, from one day to the next, is delineated with increasing clarity. Normally, exact measurements of the embryo's length can be made at least in the sixth week, and moving ultrasonic pictures can show the heart beating at a rapid rate. The length of the embryo is called the *crown-rump length* (CRL). The distance from the top of the head to the rump is measured, and the figure therefore refers to the "sitting height" of the embryo.

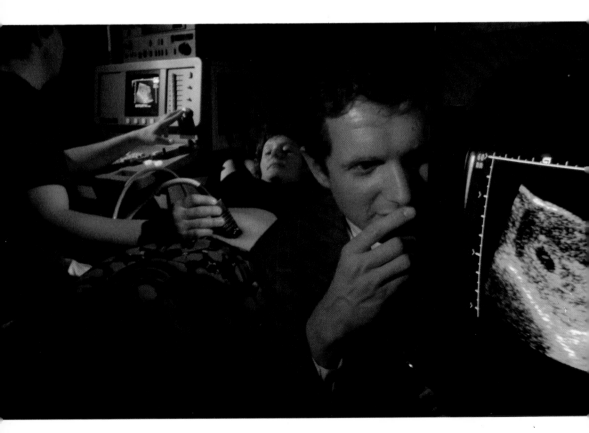

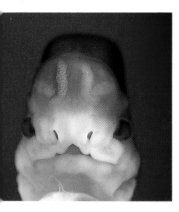

Portrait of an embryo, five and a half weeks after conception and some 14 mm (about ½ inch) long. The eyes, nose and mouth are beginning to show.

During the fifth and sixth weeks the face, trunk and limbs continue to grow. The head, which has until now been sharply inclined forward, straightens up, as does the whole embryo. There are still no skull bones, so one can see straight into the embryonic brain. Two large swellings on the forehead will become what is called the cerebrum, and three other small bulges will form various important portions of the brain. The head is almost grotesquely large compared with the rest of the body, for the embryo's growth takes place from the head downward. It is not until much later in life that the body really catches up. Even in the newborn infant the head is still roughly one-quarter of the body length, while in an adult it is only one-eighth.

The arms and legs are, as yet, extremely short, but hands and feet are starting to take shape. They look as if they are attached directly to the trunk. The hands develop considerably faster than the feet, and this difference also persists for a long time: the infant learns how to grasp objects long before it can walk. The time schedule of physical development is precisely programmed and varies little between individuals, although the genetic blueprint may vary considerably in other respects.

A father-to-be sees his baby for the first time by means of ultrasound in the seventh week of pregnancy. The embryo is then 5 weeks old and appears like a bright dot in its membrane sac. Magnified, in reality, it looks as we see it, *right*, with head, rudimentary eye, arm and hand, swimming in the fetal sac. The yolk sac, visible in the foreground, is the embryo's blood-cell factory.

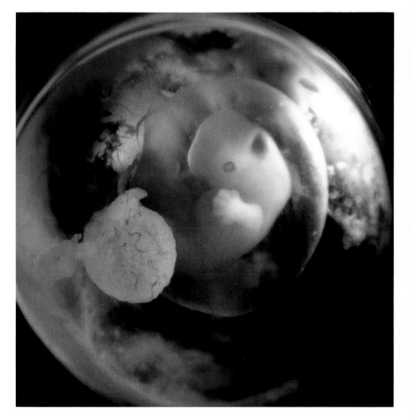

A tiny backbone

At six weeks, the spinal cord shimmers through the thin skin, but we cannot yet see much of the skeleton. Thick blood vessels—the two vertebral arteries—run down either side of the spinal cord. On its front side, vertebrae are beginning to develop and, in the back of the fragile cord, bone arches grow to surround and protect it. Meanwhile, ribs are developing as 12 horizontal rows of organized cells along the sides of the trunk. They meet in the middle, forming cartilage that later turns into bone. Between the ribs and in the body wall below the chest, muscles start to form. Over these muscles, skin forms in two layers, first a thin layer of dermis and above this layer, forming an additional sheath, the epidermis, which grows from the back forward. In this shell of skin, sweat glands and sebaceous glands soon develop like breathing holes. The skin becomes almost downy as abundant tiny, soft hairs grow from the hair follicles.

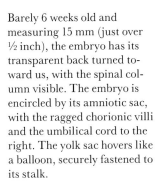

Barely 6 weeks old and measuring 15 mm (just over ½ inch), the embryo has its transparent back turned toward us, with the spinal column visible. The embryo is encircled by its amniotic sac, with the ragged chorionic villi and the umbilical cord to the right. The yolk sac hovers like a balloon, securely fastened to its stalk.

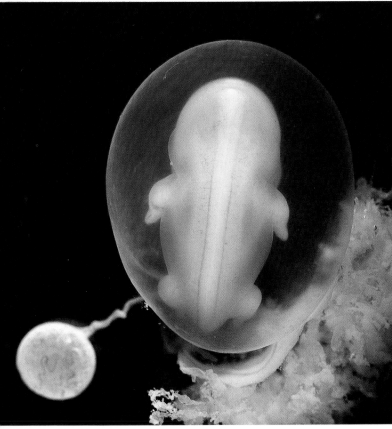

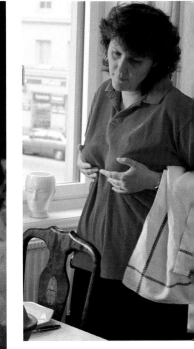

At this time, a woman's breasts feel heavy and slightly tender. Her body is undergoing increasingly radical changes.

84

Caution in taking drugs

The cells of the placenta penetrate the blood vessels of the endometrium in order to gain access to the nutrients and oxygen carried by the blood. The embryo needs more and more nourishment for its development. The placenta also serves as a filter to protect the embryo from dangerous substances in the mother's blood. This filter is usually called the "placental barrier." Though many drugs cannot pass into the embryo because they are caught in the placental barrier, others can easily pass through and enter the fetus in large quantities, causing fetal damage.

Before taking any drugs or medication, it is wise to consult with a doctor. Only those absolutely necessary to a mother's health should be considered. In many cases safe alternatives are available. Whenever possible, however, avoid drugs entirely, especially in early pregnancy, when the risk of malformations is greatest.

Six weeks after fertilization, the design for a human being begins to show results. The cells are seething with life, the heart is beating, blood is being pumped through the umbilical cord and the whole embryo is in constant motion. The embryonic heart has 140–150 fluttering beats a minute—twice as many as its mother's.

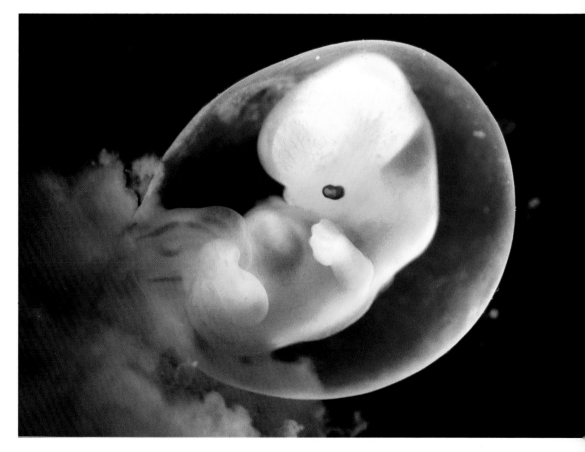

A new focus

All day long, whatever she is doing, an expectant mother's thoughts are likely to be drawn to the baby-to-be she is carrying inside her.

When she is in the eighth week, the 6-week-old embryo looks like this: a hunched little creature with dark eyes that are no more than pits in the skull; with arms, hands and legs that grow and develop from one day to the next; and with a head that is almost as large as its body.

The ball below the budding foot is the yolk sac. Here, both red blood cells and stem cells which will become the immune system's white blood cells are produced. The embryo has its own blood, separated from the mother's.

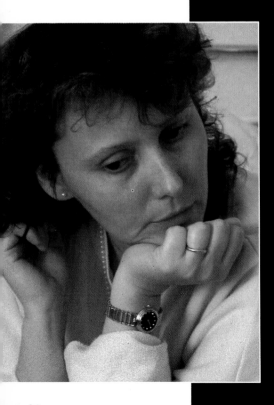

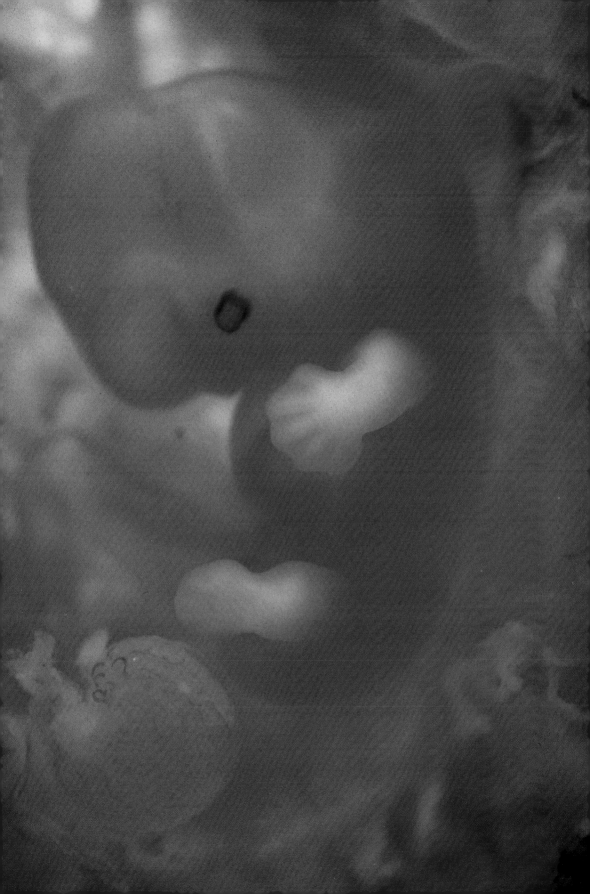

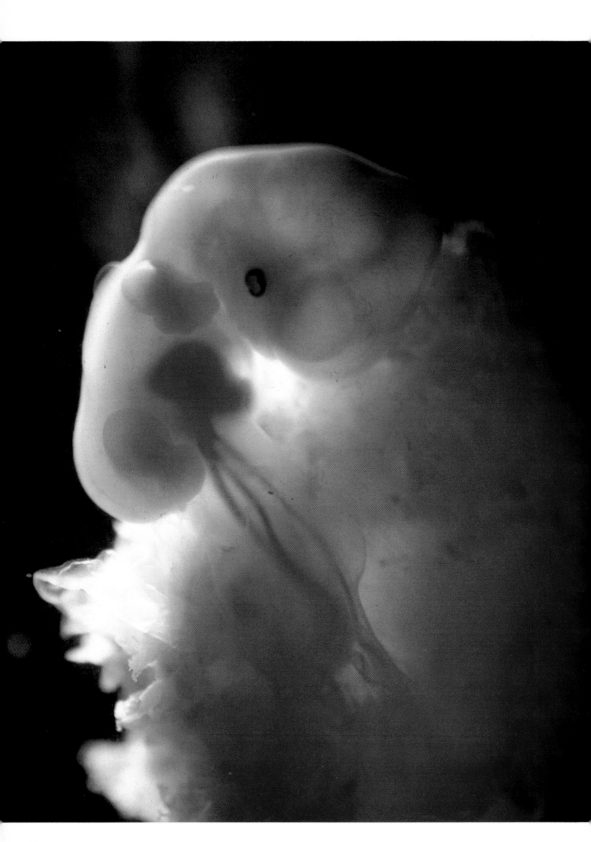

Linking two circulations

The umbilical cord is the link between the placenta and the embryo. One large blood vessel conveys oxygenated blood and nutrients to the embryo, and two vessels transport deoxygenated blood, containing waste products, back from the embryo to the placenta. The exchange of nutrients in the placenta takes place rapidly and efficiently.

The fetal blood circulation and the movement of fetal blood to and from the placenta are driven by the fetal heart, which beats rapidly—roughly twice as fast as that of the mother. The mother's circulation brings her blood to the placenta. A small portion of the oxygen is physically dissolved in the blood, and may also be released and utilized by the embryo. Hemoglobin, however, contained in the red blood cells, transports most of the oxygen in the blood. It is for this reason that the woman's blood count, i.e. the hemoglobin concentration, is monitored so carefully throughout her pregnancy.

Until birth everything that the embryo and then the fetus needs is supplied through the umbilical cord.

Every day, a great deal occurs in the embryo's development. Five and a half weeks after conception, the hand still looks like a shapeless little paddle (*left*). Three days later, we can already see the fingers (*right*).

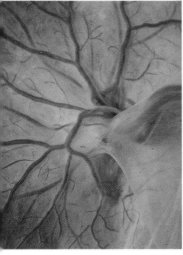

Above, embryonic and maternal bloodstreams meet—without mixing. From the placenta, blood rich in oxygen and nutrients passes to the embryo through the umbilical cord, while deoxygenated blood containing waste products passes back into the placenta.

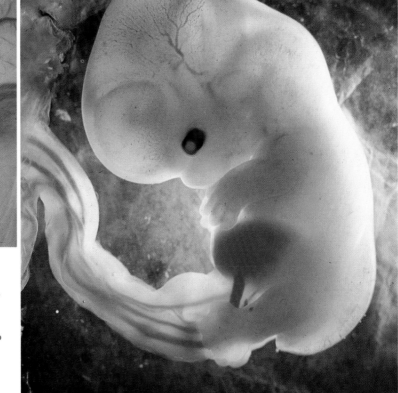

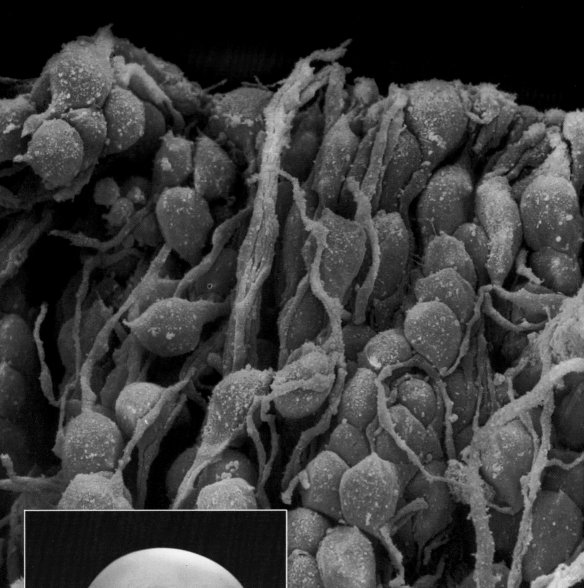

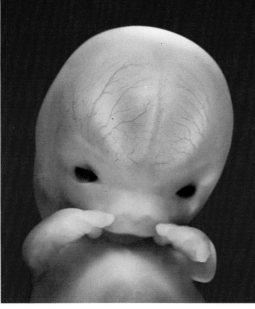

Early connections in the brain

The brain is undoubtedly one of nature's remarkable creations: cells that can react to impulses,
analyze and control behavior. As early as in the
seventh week, nerve cells in the brain have begun to
touch one another by means of projections, and some
have even become connected in primitive nerve paths.
The picture *above* shows nerve cells at this time, greatly enlarged. The rate of production is tremendous:
100,000 new nerve cells are created every minute, and
by the time the baby is born, there will be some 100
billion. *Left*, the posterior lobes of the cerebrum shimmer through the skin of the forehead.

Every organ in place

At eight weeks, the embryo is still only 4 cm (about 1½ inches) long; but inside this tiny body, all the organs are already in place. Everything to be found in a fully grown human being has already been formed. If this process has gone well, as it usually does, the risks of serious malformations are now very small, and the danger of a miscarriage also diminishes sharply. Counting from the last menstrual period, ten to eleven weeks have now elapsed.

At this point in its development, biologists start to refer to the developing being as a fetus. Previously, it has "only" been an embryo—something with excellent prospects of developing into a fetus. Despite the extraordinary progress of these two months, a great deal must still happen. The face of the fetus, the bones, hair and nails have yet to develop; most important, the brain and its functions are very undeveloped and there cannot yet be any real consciousness on the part of the fetus.

Now that the pregnancy has entered a more stable phase, with less dramatic shifts in hormone levels, the expectant woman will notice that nausea gradually subsides. The fear and risk of a miscarriage decrease, and the certainty of parenthood begins to seem more real.

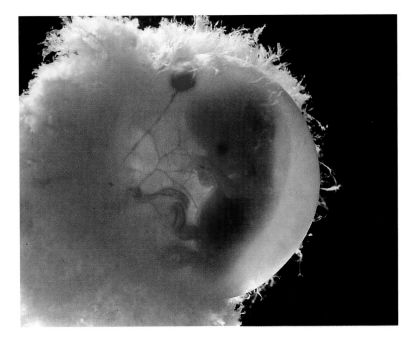

Eight weeks old, 4 cm (about 1½ inches). Weightless, the embryo lies suspended in the amniotic fluid. This fluid—with the salinity of the primeval sea—protects the embryo's delicate organs and tissues against impacts and pressure. From the placenta, the embryo's blood absorbs proteins, fat and sugar for the constant process of cell-building, as well as oxygen to fuel the process.

From embryo to fetus

Now, as it enters the eighth week after its creation in the Fallopian tube, the embryo reaches an important point in its development. The design work is complete; all its organs have been formed. From now on, the embryo must grow, develop what has been created, refine its functions and test its systems. The embryo graduates to a new stage and becomes a fetus.

The fetus now weighs roughly 13 g (less than ½ ounce), excluding the auxiliary organs. In 50 days, the embryo has been transformed from a single cell into many millions, all precisely programmed for their specific tasks. How this fantastic development is governed in detail is still, in many respects, a mystery.

In every cell of this eye, this hand and these fingers, there are about 100,000 genes. How does the cell know that it is to become part of the cornea, the lens, the vitreous body, the retina or the optical nerve? How does it know which genes are to be used at each crucial moment, and which are to be excluded?

The mother—the woman bearing the budding life and wondering at everything that is happening in her body—need not concern herself with these questions. Development follows a pattern laid down in the dawn of prehistory, and her contribution is to live in such a way that this pattern of development is not disrupted.

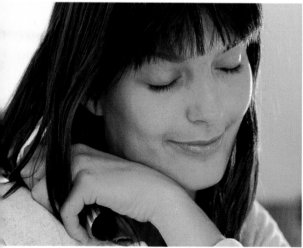

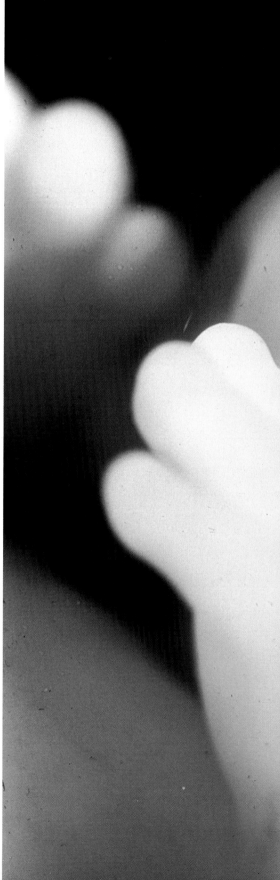

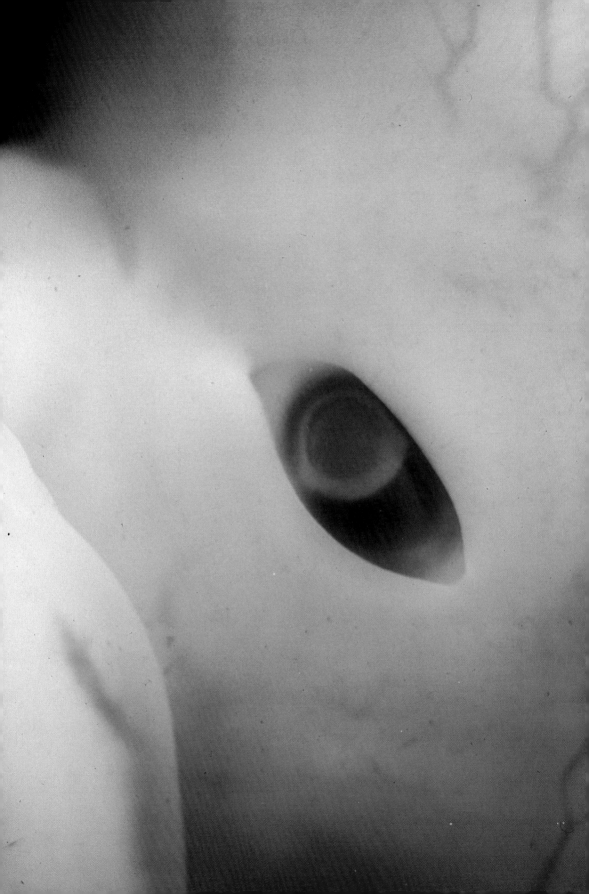

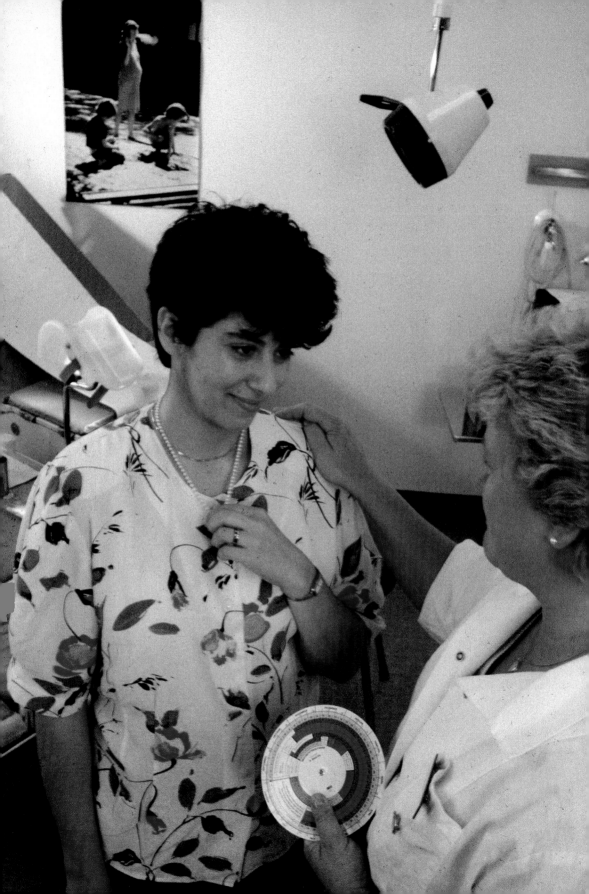

Early Pregnancy

For most women, it is a heady feeling to know that a baby is on the way. For others, questions are raised: Can I, and should I, stay pregnant? Around the world, somewhat over one-quarter of pregnant women answer these questions in the negative and opt for abortion instead. The earlier an abortion is carried out, the less complicated the procedure. Within the first three months, an abortion is technically very simple, and usually the woman can leave the clinic or hospital after a few hours. In certain countries, drugs are becoming available which, taken in the early weeks, lower levels of progesterone and bring on an abortion similar to a heavy menstrual period. Whatever the regulations surrounding abortion in any particular country, or the procedure, the decision to terminate pregnancy is difficult for a woman, and very often also for the man concerned.

But when a pregnancy is desired, women greet the news in a mood of happy anticipation, bursting with questions and thoughts. The first medical appointment will be with a doctor, or in some cases, a midwife. This will take place at the doctor's office or at an obstetrical (antenatal) clinic. It is essential for the doctor to be informed whether the woman suffers from any illness, or has in the past, and about any medication she is taking. Heart, liver and kidney diseases may affect the prospects of both fetus and mother. The same applies to diabetes, in which the mother's need of insulin almost always increases during pregnancy. A family history, including the incidence of genetic diseases, disabilities and of twins or other multiple births is also taken.

Maternal age is an important factor in pregnancy. Though women can conceive and give birth right up to the age of about 50, once a woman has passed the age of 35 or so, the risks of certain chromosome defects in the fetus increase. This applies particularly to Down syndrome. A woman in her late thirties or over should seriously consider having fetal diagnosis performed.

The most common test is amniocentesis, carried out by extracting a sample of amniotic fluid via the mother's abdominal wall and examining the chromosomes in the fetal cells.

For the mother-to-be expecting her first child, visiting the clinic or doctor's office for the very first time is a momentous occasion. She is bursting with questions, full of happiness and anticipation—but at the same time a little uncertain. The situation is, after all, so new.

When can I expect to feel the first fetal movements? What is the estimated date of delivery? These days, the doctor or the midwife can give some fairly reliable answers, as well as needed reassurance.

There are reasons both for and against amniocentesis, and the advisability of this test and others, such as chorionic villus sampling (CVS), which can also detect chromosomal abnormalities and is done earlier than amniocentesis, should be thoroughly discussed. If there are concerns about neural tube defects such as spina bifida, a test known as an alpha-fetoprotein test is done, using a blood sample.

Previous pregnancies

It is also important to discuss any earlier pregnancies. It may, perhaps, have been by cesarean section last time: in that case, what was the reason? How did it go? Formerly, the belief was "once a cesarean, always a cesarean"—an old wives' tale that has fallen into disrepute. If the cesarean section is carried out because the woman's pelvis is too narrow, it will of course have to be repeated next time, since the woman's pelvic canal does not expand with age. But the reason for performing the cesarean may also have been that the fetal blood supply was suddenly curtailed in the course of delivery. The umbilical cord may have been constricted, and this kind of complication does not necessarily recur. A vaginal delivery may usually therefore be planned, even if the mother has already undergone a cesarean. Other factors, such as the nature of the incision in the previous cesarean, will affect the decision.

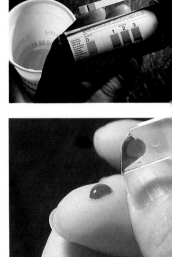

Blood samples from the finger or fold of the arm and urine samples are taken during pregnancy to check the blood count, the presence of sugar and protein in the urine, and other variables of particular importance in pregnancy.

Laboratory tests

After the discussion, several laboratory tests are done. A sample of the mother-to-be's urine is taken, to see whether protein or sugar is leaking out via the kidneys. Normally, this should not be the case, but pregnancy imposes strains on the kidneys and urinary tract.

Several blood samples are routinely taken to ascertain the blood group and whether the woman is immune to German measles, and also to determine the hemoglobin content of the blood—a measure of the blood's capacity to transport oxygen. This capacity is very important in enabling the fetus to receive enough oxygen for its metabolism and growth. A low hemoglobin value is usually caused by iron deficiency. On the first visit, tests are also carried out for syphilis and sometimes gonorrhea and chlamydia.

Physical examination

In many cases, a physician will choose to do a pelvic examination. This starts with the insertion of an instrument called a speculum into the vagina, enabling the doctor or midwife to see and examine the vaginal membranes and the cervix itself. When a woman is pregnant, the cervix has a distinctive, slightly swollen appearance and the color of the membrane is somewhat purplish. A "Pap test" (cervical smear) is carried out to check for cervical cancer, depending upon when this was last done.

Sometimes the doctor will feel the uterus with one hand on the woman's stomach and two fingers deep inside the vagina. An experienced obstetrician can immediately determine whether the size of the uterus corresponds to the "gestational age" (the duration of the pregnancy). These days, ultrasound scans can give more accurate information. The physician may also measure the pelvis, to estimate the size of the passageway through which the baby must navigate at birth.

The medical examination also includes a thorough check of the breasts, which have usually become enlarged and tender. The breast tissue may be quite lumpy. During any part of this examination, the woman should feel free to ask questions, for this is an excellent time to learn more about her anatomy.

Sometimes around the 12th or 13th week, counted from the onset of the last menstrual period, sometimes earlier, the pregnant woman usually goes for her first medical examination. The doctor may perform a Pap test (cervical smear) on a cell sample from the cervix. The doctor may then feel the uterus, with one hand on the woman's stomach and two fingers deep inside her vagina.

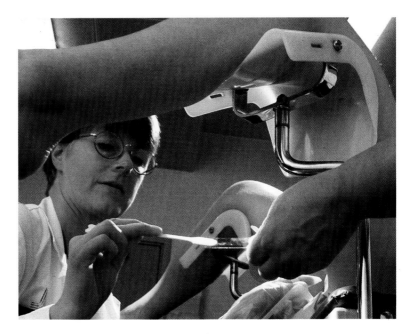

When is the baby due?

This question is, to many women, the most important one to have answered on the first visit, and it is always discussed. The average pregnancy lasts 280 days, but it is also known that deviations of 14 days in either direction are fairly common (95 percent of all babies are born between the 266th and the 294th day). The conventional method of calculation begins with the first day of the last menstrual period, to which nine months and seven days are added. If the woman has menstrual cycles exceeding 28 days, ovulation will be later and it may be necessary to add one or two weeks. These days, ultrasound scans provide fairly accurate information about the stage of pregnancy and have replaced more speculative calculations.

Overly rigid expectations as to the date of delivery on the part of the patient or doctor can be harmful. In the highly scheduled modern world, birth is one event which cannot, and should not, be tightly controlled. Attempts to induce labor can result in ineffective contractions, difficult and protracted labor and the birth of a baby who would, perhaps, have benefited greatly from remaining in the uterus for another week or two. Also, the drugs which are sometimes administered during childbirth to stimulate contractions are not entirely harmless to the baby and must be used sparingly.

On later visits to the doctor or maternity antenatal clinic, the distance between the upper edge of the pubic bone and the top curve of the uterus (the symphysis-fundus measurement) may be ascertained with a tape measure, yet another way of monitoring fetal growth.

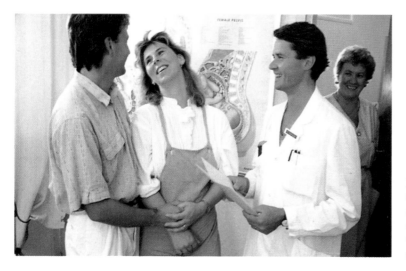

Heartening news: after the first examination, the doctor can usually sum up that everything appears normal. The woman's worry and tension are superseded by relief and joy.

Diet during pregnancy

The mother's "growth" is monitored by her weight. During the first three months (first trimester) of pregnancy, weight gain is seldom a problem since most women experience slight nausea. However, when this nausea diminishes in due course, many women develop an unusually keen appetite, probably because their blood-sugar level falls more rapidly after a meal. This is due to the fact that the fetus is gradually consuming ever larger amounts of nourishment.

Many stories are told about the *pica syndrome*—the pregnant woman's almost irresistible craving for some particular kind of food, a certain fruit or sometimes strange foods such as licorice and oysters, or even newsprint or mortar. These cravings are probably due to some deficiency in the normal diet.

A weight increase of roughly 12 kilograms (25–30 pounds) by the end of pregnancy is an optimum goal. A very large weight gain and obesity in general have been associated with complications at birth. Food that is nourishing at other stages of life is appropriate during pregnancy as well. However, the pregnant woman should eat more often than other people, and choose a variety of fresh, vitamin-rich, rather than high-calorie foods. Fruits and vegetables, a variety of whole grains, high-protein food such as fish, eggs, low-fat dairy products, lean meat or beans are important. Dietary supplements of iron and vitamins are often prescribed, at least in late pregnancy. New parents-to-be often feel highly motivated to change their eating habits and prepare healthier meals.

Many pregnant women experience an unlimited craving for a certain kind of food. After childbirth, the woman herself may find it difficult to understand this fixation on food with a particular flavor.

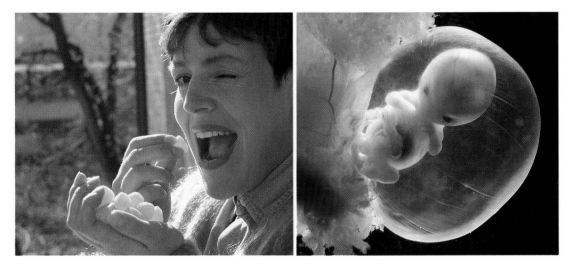

Feminine hygiene

The risk of an infection spreading up through the cervix to the uterus and affecting the fetus is very small in a normal pregnancy. A shower—preferably hand-held—makes feminine hygiene easier. Soap should not be used inside the vagina: the suds may be difficult to rinse away properly, and can lead to irritation. Swimming in clean water is not harmful. Sunbathing should be undertaken in moderation. It is inadvisable for a pregnant woman to become severely overheated, and the sun may also produce unattractive brown patches on the skin, since the hormonal changes of pregnancy also affect pigmentation.

Vaccinations and infectious diseases

Most vaccinations are less advisable during pregnancy and some are downright dangerous. They should therefore be avoided. One should preferably refrain from traveling to countries where the risk of infection is great. Rubella (German measles) is a dangerous infection in early pregnancy and can result in fetal impairment. Even if the illness does not manifest itself in an unmistakable rash, blood tests repeated every few weeks can establish with certainty whether one has become infected. If the woman suspects this to be the case, she should therefore contact her doctor or the clinic. Since the defects caused by rubella can be so severe, an infected woman may not wish to continue her pregnancy. For women who are not pregnant, a vaccine is available. Women should also contact the doctor or clinic for other infections, such as severe colds, diarrhea with stomach pain, high temperatures and skin rashes. In treating such illnesses during pregnancy, it is important to know which medicines may be taken without jeopardizing fetal health.

Intercourse

A warm, loving relationship is more important than ever during pregnancy. It can be a time of growing closeness for a couple and there is generally no reason to avoid intercourse. If the woman has previously had a miscarriage or if anything untoward—such as bleeding or premature uterine contractions—occurs, the woman should discuss the situation with her doctor or midwife. Asking about this subject is nothing to be embarrassed about but, rather, entirely natural and important.

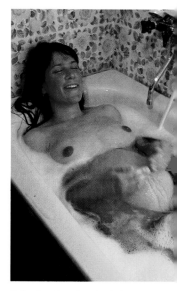

Relaxing in a hot bath is particularly enjoyable if one's back is aching and stiff.

Alcohol and tobacco

In recent years, an intensive debate has been under way concerning the harmful impact of alcohol on the fetus. The findings of large-scale surveys have shown that heavy drinkers have exposed their babies to serious malformation risks, both during the early embryonic stage and in the latter phase of fetal development. In particular, eyes and vision are easily damaged by alcohol. This probably does not mean that a single glass of beer or wine during pregnancy is harmful. However, as with any other substances that pass into the baby's bloodstream, caution is the wisest course. Regular consumption is definitely not advisable.

Smoking is also dangerous, since the oxygen-bearing capacity of the woman's blood deteriorates as a result of smoking. Nicotine and carbon monoxide from smoking affect the fetus, since these substances can pass through the placental barrier into the fetal bloodstream. Many clinics and doctors can suggest programs to help women give up smoking. Those who do not wish to, or feel they cannot, stop smoking during pregnancy may perhaps be persuaded to reduce their cigarette consumption drastically. During this period, a smokeless environment at the workplace is more important than ever, especially since nausea during pregnancy is often exacerbated by tobacco smoke.

Smoking always affects the blood circulation, since nicotine causes the blood vessels to contract. Every puff on a cigarette constricts the flow of blood in the umbilical cord, subjecting the fetus to stress. Babies born to women who are heavy smokers almost always weigh less at birth than they would have if the mother had stopped smoking at the beginning of her pregnancy.

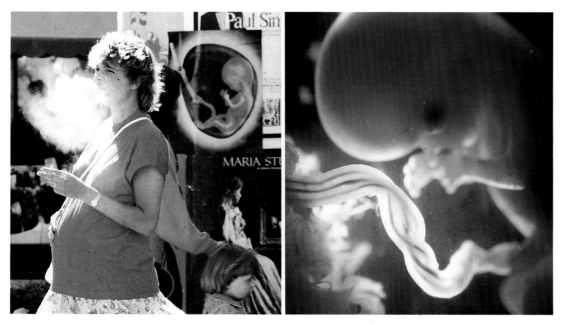

Live as usual

Pregnancy is not an illness and should not be regarded as such. Most women can work as usual until a few weeks before delivery. Back trouble and difficulty in retaining urine when the fetus kicks against the bladder are ailments that may cause problems at work toward the end of pregnancy. However, women often feel better psychologically at work, compared with staying at home, where they may become more aware of a number of minor pains that are common in late pregnancy.

Employer's responsibility

Certain jobs may involve increased risk. Pregnant women who work in radiology departments should be transferred in order to avoid the slightest risk of being exposed to radiation. The same applies to women whose work involves toxic substances in industry or cell toxins at hospitals. Although nearly all researchers agree that computer screens do not emit radiation dangerous to the fetus, other factors, such as the stress to which computer operators are exposed, may perhaps constitute a risk. In later pregnancy, heavy lifting should be avoided. Many of these risk factors, such as radiation or toxins, are potentially dangerous to other workers as well. In such cases, concerns for safety should apply to the whole work force, rather than become a reason to ban women from certain jobs.

A healthy work environment becomes even more important during pregnancy. Toxic substances can damage the sensitive embryo at an early stage, and at a later stage, the expectant mother should, of course, avoid lifting heavy objects.

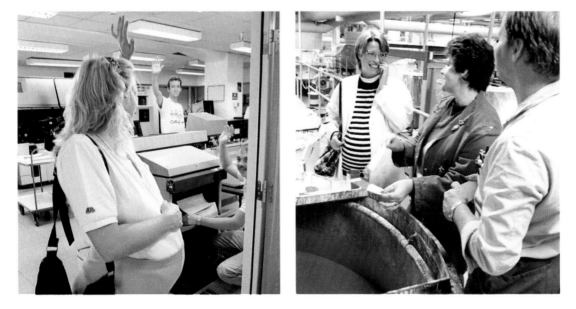

Ultrasound

For more than 20 years, our hospitals have been equipped with ultrasound devices. Radiology departments were the first to be attracted by this technology, which often yielded as much information as X rays. But unlike X rays, ultrasound waves appear to be entirely harmless. Nowadays, most departments of obstetrics and maternity hospitals have access to this technique. Ultrasound waves have such a high frequency—more than 20,000 cycles per second—that they cannot be detected by the human ear. The sound waves pass through the body, and when they meet tissue of a different density, part of the sound is reflected back as an echo; it is these echoes that form the pictures on the screen.

The first ultrasound machines produced still pictures of the fetus, but in the last decade, moving images in sharp focus have enhanced the technique's potential. Aided by a technician's or doctor's explanation, the mother can see the tiny embryo on the screen from the fifth week onward. She can see the little heart beating, and later in pregnancy, clear fetal movements are also visible.

One important item of information given on the ultrasound screen is the position of the placenta in the uterus. The presence of twins (or more) is also revealed at an early stage by this technique. In many parts of the world, every woman is offered at least one ultrasound scan during her pregnancy. This is usually carried out in the 16th or 17th week, when the scan can give a good indication of any fetal malformations present. If these are grave, it is still not too late for abortion. However, there may be some uncertainty even among experts, and in such cases, the parents may be confronted by an extremely difficult decision.

A more positive side of the technique is that, using ultrasound, surgeons can perform life-saving operations on the fetus while it is still inside the uterus. In the future, operations of this kind will undoubtedly become both more numerous and more widespread. Ultrasound equipment with an additional device that functions in a manner reminiscent of a sonic-depth finder (a Doppler ultrasound) may also be used to measure such variables as the fetal blood supply—a measurement that may be crucial in late pregnancy. At that point, the question often arises as to whether this fetus will thrive best if it remains and develops inside the uterus, or will benefit more from leaving the uterus.

First sight of the baby

Seeing one's unborn child in the uterus is an indescribable experience, as awesome as Earth seen from the moon, or Jupiter's Great Red Spot. Seen on the ultrasound screen the fetus waves, kicks and swivels in the amniotic sac. And we can hear its rapid heartbeat.

Bottom: until the 16th week, the whole fetus is visible on the screen of the ultrasound device; later on, the images show only parts of its body. The pictures are a visual translation of the ultrasound echo registered by the device.

The ultrasound scan can provide answers to questions on the duration of pregnancy, the size of the fetus and whether the woman is expecting twins. It can also reveal certain abnormalities. Ultrasound scans have assumed an increasingly important role in fetal diagnostics.

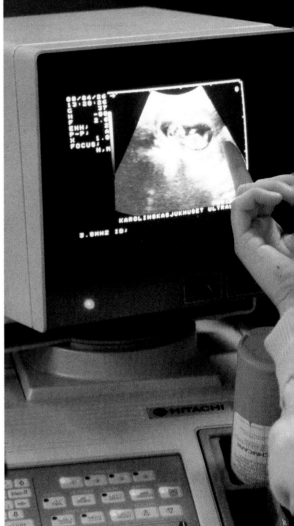

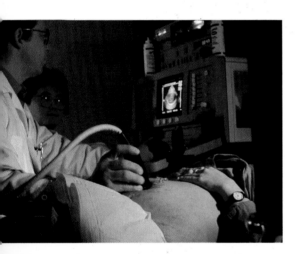

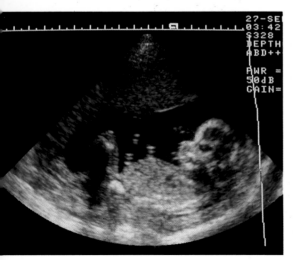

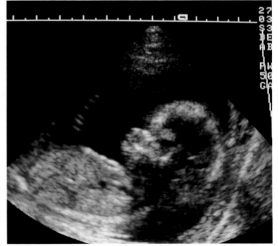

104

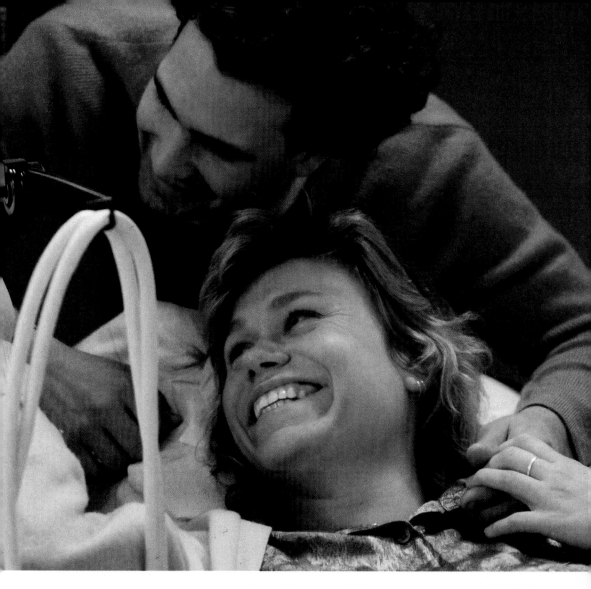

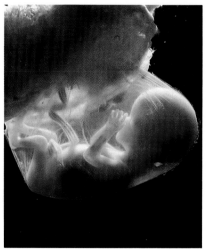

Left, a fetus in the 16th week of pregnancy, visualized through ultrasound. *Right*, a fetus of the same age, in a photograph.

The mother-to-be can obtain a copy of the ultrasound image—a cherished first portrait of her baby to put in the family album. A few years later, the subject of the picture will greatly appreciate it as well.

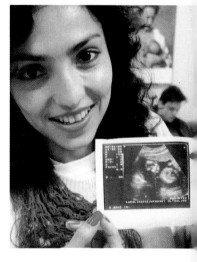

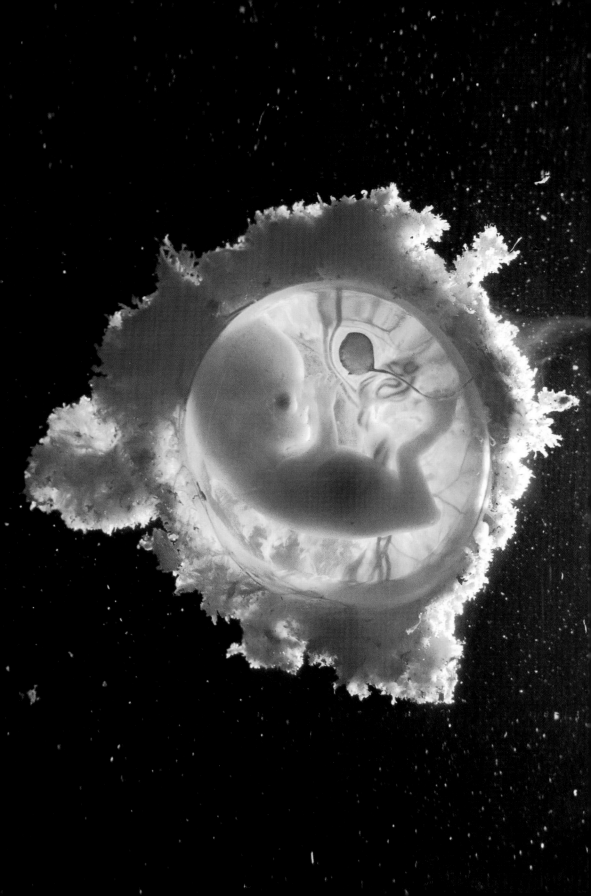

Fetal Development

In the *third month*, the fetus is well established in the uterus, its organs and organ systems are becoming interconnected, and the brain and the sensory organs are beginning to play an important part in these developments. In the placenta, all the hormones needed for the rest of the pregnancy are now being produced. The placenta is also responsible for the entire interchange of nutrients to and waste products from the fetus.

During the embryonic stage, blood cells are formed in the yolk sac, which has no other task in the body. Inside the sac, the stem cells that in due course give rise to differentiated white blood cells also take shape. These blood cells form the basis of the fetal immune system, which protects it against infections. As early as the 11th week, the yolk sac has ceased to serve its purpose; thereafter, blood cells are formed in the liver and the spleen. The fetus's own bone marrow soon also starts producing blood cells. The white blood cells from the bone marrow must then proceed to the lymph glands and the thymus for further development.

The fetus is not normally exposed to infections, since most bacteria and viruses cannot pass through the placental filter. Among the exceptions are rubella and syphilis. The remarkable fact is that a 5-month-old fetus can already partly defend itself against infections by means of its own immune system.

Mankind is a newcomer to the universe, and this 3-month-old fetus may be seen as a symbol of our advent — a space traveler in his capsule, complete with lifeline. The ragged halo is the chorionic sac, which adheres to the placenta.

Most expectant mothers can exercise freely throughout pregnancy: jogging, skiing cross-country or doing keep-fit exercises as she wishes.

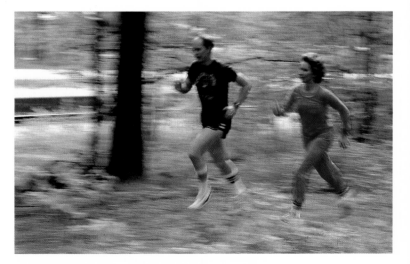

A warm shelter

Ten or eleven weeks old and measuring 3–3½ cm (about 1⅓ inches) from crown to rump, the fetus still enjoys ample space and is warm and comfortable in the amniotic fluid. The temperature is 37.5°C (99.5°F) — somewhat higher than that of the mother, who in turn is slightly warmer than before she became pregnant.

What can the fetus do? Its body jerks and moves, it hiccups and it flexes its arms and tiny legs, testing its newfound abilities.

The yolk sac, the ball-shaped blood-cell factory, to the left in the photograph, has served its purpose by the 11th week, when the liver, spleen and bone marrow take over production. Its stem will soon become detached. The drawing *below*, which is life-size, indicates the situation in the growing uterus, the neck of which (the cervix) is blocked with a plug of mucus as protection against invading bacteria.

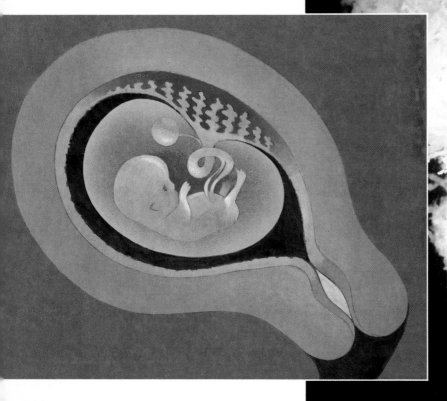

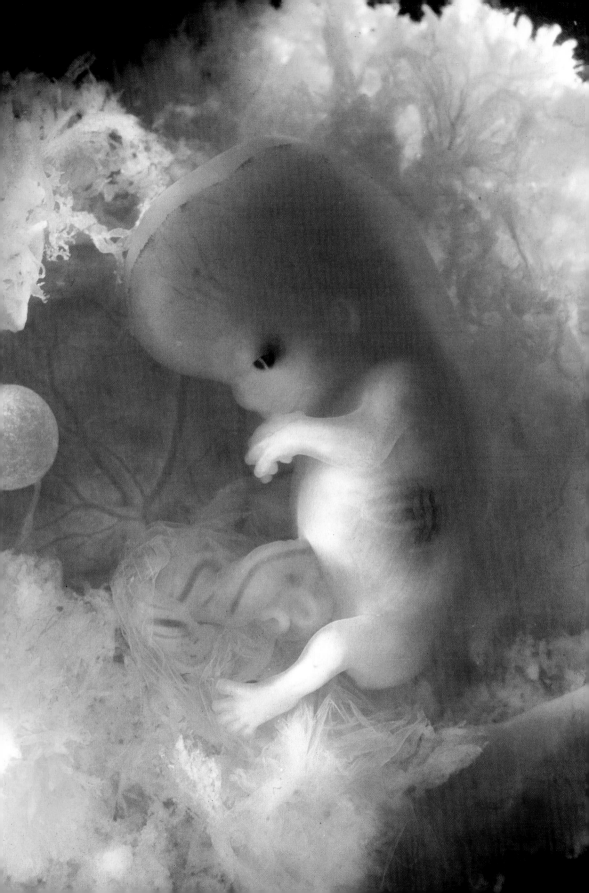

A human being in the making

During the fourth month, the fetus grows from 5 cm to over 10 cm (about 2 to 4 inches). Its weight is not yet impressive: approximately 20 g (under one ounce) at the age of 11 weeks. The proportions of the fetus have become more "human," but the head is still disproportionately large—roughly one-third of the entire body length. The face is developing more and more and by the age of 11 to 12 weeks is beginning to look recognizably human.

To form the face, five outgrowths, known as "processes," emerge and join under the thin skin. The first proceeds down between the eyes and ends in a "bay" on either side—the future nostrils—thus forming the nose and the middle of the upper lip. Two other processes appear under the eyes and form the cheeks and the sides of the upper lip. The last two grow under the mouth, fusing to form the lower lip and the chin. Muscles now become attached to this framework, enabling the face to move. Facial expressions—frowning, lips that open or shut, a turn of the head—begin to appear, but our interpretations of their meaning are still mere guesses.

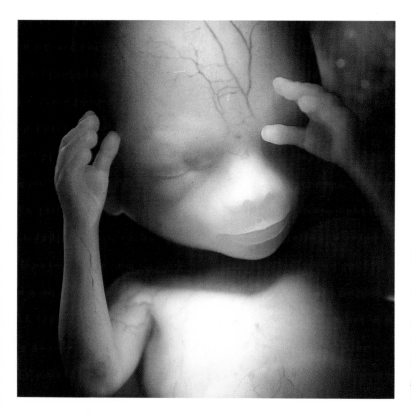

Fifteen weeks, 10 cm (4 inches). Now the facial features are being modeled: the forehead is growing, with the threadlike blood vessel fully visible under the transparent skin. The eyelids have closed and will not open again until the fetus is 7 months old. The nail beds are appearing on the fingers, and the arms have grown long enough for the hands to grasp each other.

Creation proceeds apace, silently, in the shelter of the placenta—which not only provides food and removes waste products but also shields the fetus with hormones that prevent a new ovulation and menstrual period. The fetus is becoming more and more lively—turning its head, moving its face and making breathing movements.

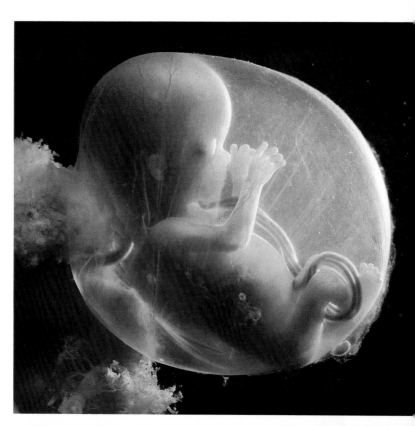

The mother is now beginning to have difficulty in doing up her skirt, and her children are becoming ever more interested in knowing what is going on in her swelling abdomen.

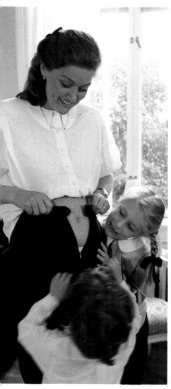

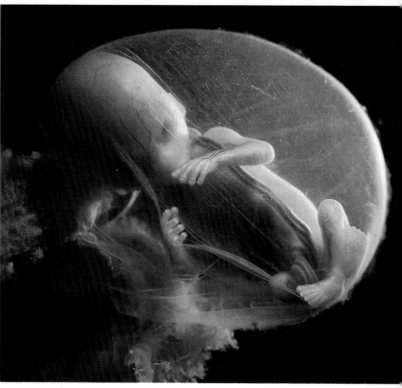

Eyes and vision

The development of the eye is a remarkable example of the close interaction between the developing brain and the thin skin on the embryo's temples. First of all, the forebrain issues a hollow stalk on either side. The end of the stalk thickens, forming a small sphere. When this meets the inside of the skin it turns inward on itself like a cup. The base of the cup becomes the fundus or back of the eyeball, and the skin surface covering it the retina. Inside the cup, the skin cells then form a lens and a cornea. On the front of the lens, an iris grows inward from the edges. Finally, the surrounding skin folds over to form two eyelids. The eye is complete.

Can the fetus see inside the uterus? We do not know, but we know that the eyes are sensitive to light. If a doctor looks inside the uterus at a mid-term fetus, using a fetoscope with a light attachment, the fetus tries to shield its eyes from the light with its hands.

All visual impressions must be read and interpreted by the primary visual area in the brain, located farthest back at the base of the skull. Long nerve-paths extend from each eye, crossing before they reach the visual cortex of the brain. Here, impressions are sorted into light and dark, and a variety of colors and shapes, from which whole pictorial images are constructed. The newborn baby first learns to recognize pictures that recur frequently. Above all, a mother's or father's face is an interesting object on which to gaze, while strangers' faces are more difficult to interpret and therefore unsettling at first.

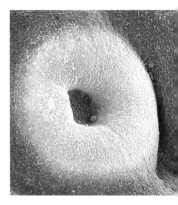

The eye has long been considered the mirror of the soul. As such, its beginnings are modest (*above*, 30 days). By week 13, the eye is well developed and the lids close for several months (*right*).

5 weeks

6½ weeks

8 weeks

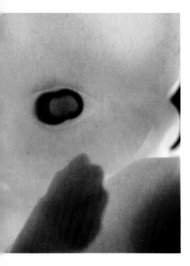

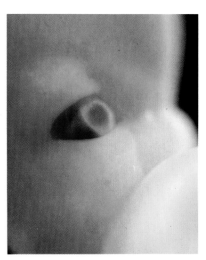

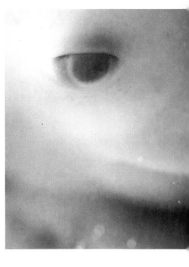

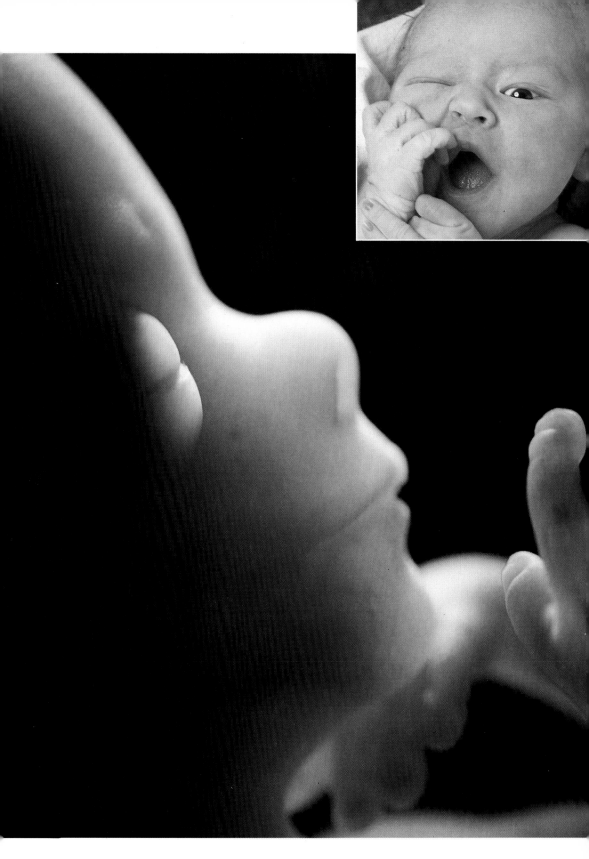

Ears and hearing

A fetus begins to react to sound sometime between early in the fourth month and the fifth, and is both stimulated and irritated by sounds. The ear itself is formed from three components, developing from three different directions during the actual construction process. From the embryo's thin skin, a hollow forms on either side of the hindbrain. This eventually becomes the inner ear, containing the auditory and balance organs. Slightly later, the outer ear develops, with the auditory canal and the outer side of the eardrum. The intermediate portion — the middle ear, with its auditory bones (hammer, anvil and stirrup) — develops as a bulge from the pharynx.

Infections such as German measles in the mother's body during the critical weeks when the ears are being formed may result in malformations and hearing impairment. As the pregnancy proceeds, the fetus can hear more and more sound variations, and its brain can interpret them. Thus, the fetus by no means lives in a silent world. In particular, the rumblings of the mother's stomach and intestines, the sound of blood flowing through her blood vessels and her heart beat are noises that penetrate the uterus from outside. Singing to one's unborn child is a common recommendation and a tradition in many cultures. Most specialists in this area consider that the mother's voice and pulse are impressions of importance to the fetus. A newborn baby, for instance, will turn to a female — in preference to a male — voice.

If the father is musical, he can start communicating with the fetus as early as in the fifth month, when it starts reacting to sounds. And if the mother sings to her unborn child before birth, she may later find that the newborn baby recognizes the tune.

The outer ear begins to take shape in the eighth week, but does not resemble a fully formed ear until the fifth month. *Right*, a fetus 15 weeks old.

8 weeks

4 months

5 months

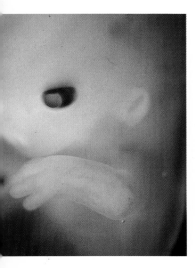

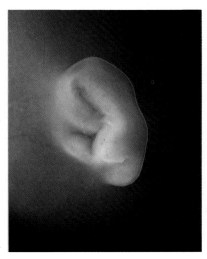

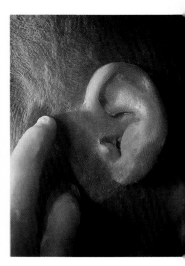

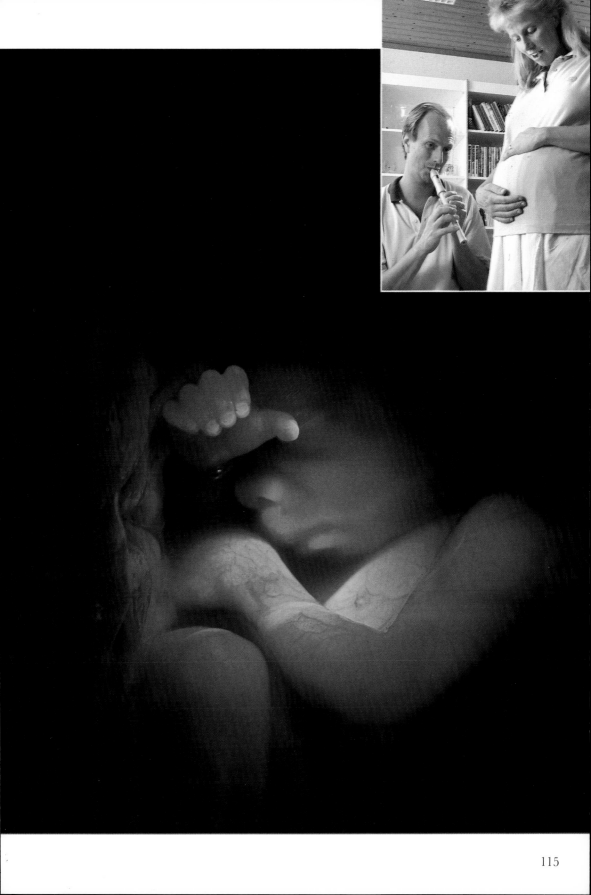

Hand and foot

Four weeks after conception, a clear stripe is formed along either side of the trunk, from the rudimentary shoulder to what will become the hip. The stripe is composed of cells from the middle germ (cell) layer. In the fifth week, two small, protruding buds are visible. The buds are slightly flattened and reminiscent of a seal's flipper. Each bud develops an edge that soon thickens into a ridge. The ridge now takes the lead, issuing instructions to the connective tissue to make preparations for the upper arm, forearm and hand, or the thigh, lower leg and foot, respectively. The hand is formed before the foot, and the arms and legs become elongated later, in due course assuming the usual proportions. In the third to the fourth month, the hand can already grasp and the foot can kick, although the kicks are still too small and weak for a mother to notice them.

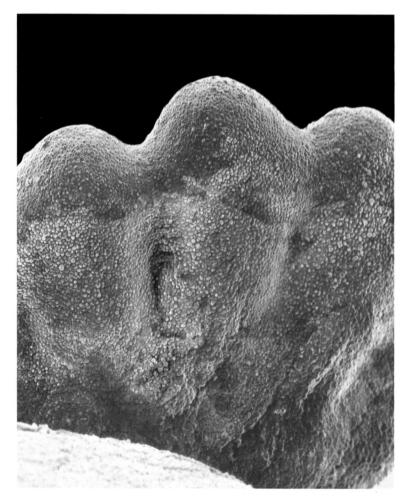

Formation of the fingers

Six weeks after the fertilization of the ovum, the embryonic hand is taking shape and the rudiments of fingers are visible. The tissue between them regresses and dies. The epithelial cells of the skin are sharply delineated. *Right,* some eight months later, the grasping reflex has developed.

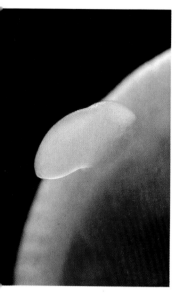

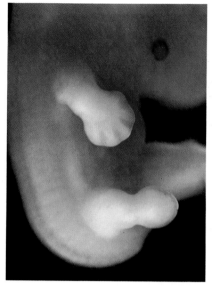

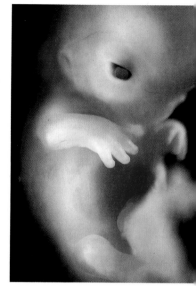

The arm bud begins to protrude from the trunk as early as in the third or fourth week. Two weeks later, the hand is clearly in advance of the foot in its development, and the finger buds are visible. In the 11th week (*far right, above*), five tiny fingers may be discerned on each hand; and in week 17 (*right*), the nails may be seen.

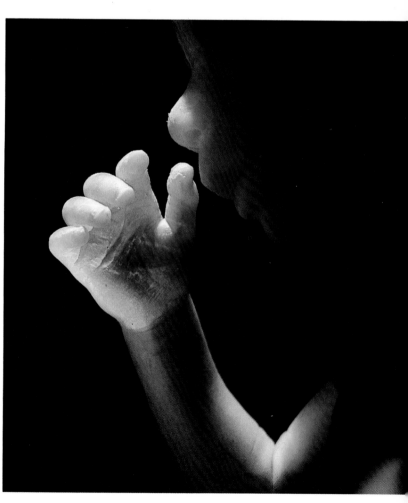

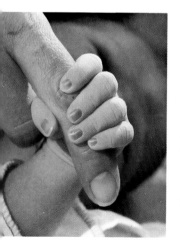

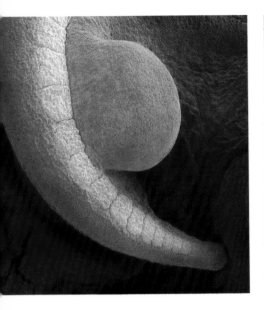

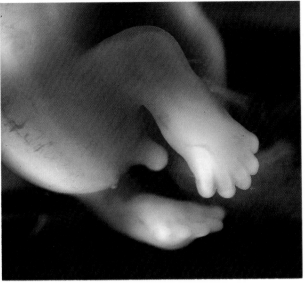

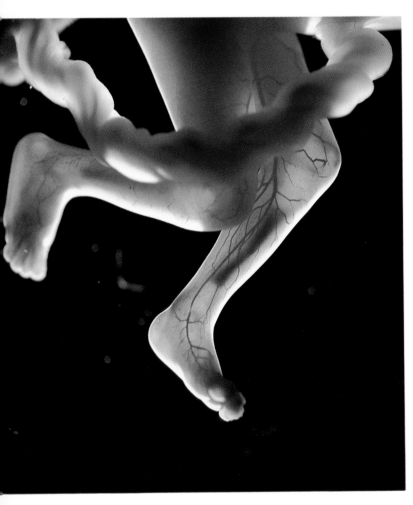

The foot

The tail is a link with our animal past, and it is lost as early as in the seventh or eighth fetal week, but we retain several small, shrunken tail vertebrae even after birth.

Above left, the tail and the foot and leg buds in week four may be seen. *Above right*, in week nine, both foot and toes have developed.

Four months old, 16 cm (about 6½ inches) long. When the feet and toes are partially developed, it is the leg's turn to grow. Through the thin skin, the now ossified long bone in the middle portion of the lower leg is visible, while the rest of the skeleton is still composed of cartilage. The spiral shape of the umbilical cord is caused by the fact that the two arteries and the vein are longer than the sheath in which they are contained—an ingenious safety device for lively fetuses!

Bones

The tremendous development and growth undergone by the fetus inside the uterine cavity mean that its body must be highly malleable throughout. Cartilage is softer and more plastic than bone, and it therefore forms the initial structure. This cartilage will be partially converted into bone later. The newborn infant's bones are still very soft and pliable. The flexible skull bones may incur large indentations in the course of birth. Such changes are repaired spontaneously and swiftly. Collarbones and upper arms may also sometimes break during birth if the passage is unduly narrow. Unlike fractures in adults, nothing usually needs to be done about these breaks; they heal without the slightest scar or trace, and the babies concerned do not appear to suffer particularly.

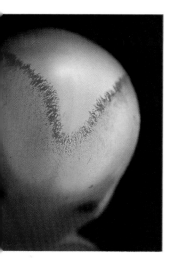

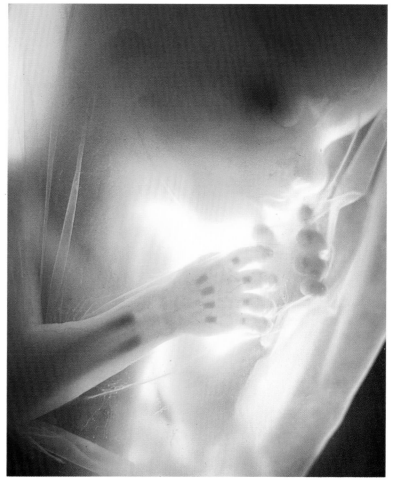

Eight weeks old, the fetus is changing at tremendous speed. Numerous blood vessels are growing, V-shaped, over the crown, but soft boneless patches (the fontanel) remain right up to the age of about 2 years. During birth, the skull bones may be forced to overlap in order for the head to pass through the birth canal. *Right*, we can see the bone shafts in the hand and arm of the 12-week-old fetus.

Hair

The first signs of hair appear in the third month. They start as a suggestion of whiskers, and are later replaced by the hair called *lanugo*, which covers the whole body and forms intriguing patterns on the skin. The patterns are due to the oblique lie of the hair follicles, which follow the connective-tissue fibers in the layer of the skin beneath the epidermis.

In the fourth to fifth month, the hairs on the fetus's head and in the eyebrows become slightly coarser, and are colored by special pigment cells. The lanugo is shed and disappears before birth, and we still do not know its actual purpose. The tiny hairs may possibly serve to retain the protective skin ointment (the vernix caseosa) that is formed from the sebaceous glands around the hair follicles. This waxy substance provides good protection against skin infections and makes the baby slippery during birth. Some of the vernix caseosa comes off the fetus's body and is mixed with the amniotic fluid, which becomes cloudy toward the end of pregnancy.

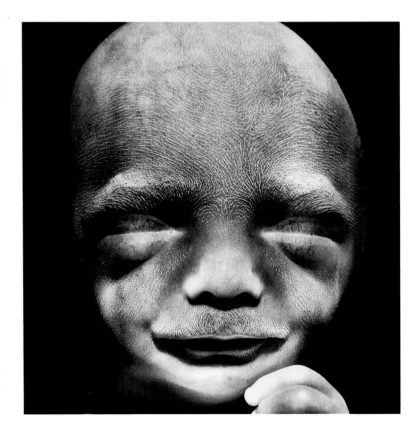

Why is the fetus furry?

Right: barely 6 months old, the fetus is covered all over by downy hair. Is this furry covering a residual link with the beginning of human evolution or does the hair serve a purpose—for example, in holding the waxy vernix which protects the fetus's skin? By the time of birth it has disappeared, and only the hair on the head remains.

As we see *left*, the matted lanugo forms interesting patterns owing to the oblique way the hair roots are positioned in the skin. They follow the connective-fiber threads in the corium, the layer between the epidermis and the dermis.

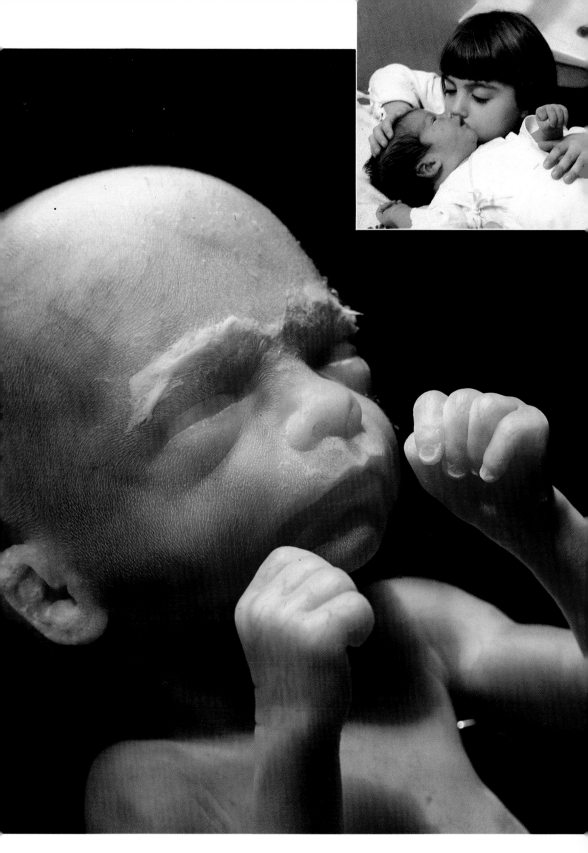

Boy or girl?

The baby's sex is determined at the moment of fertilization. During the first few months of fetal development, it is impossible to tell boys and girls apart with the naked eye: the sex glands and organs look exactly the same. Between the legs a small bud develops that later becomes the boy's penis or the girl's clitoris. Two swellings emerge, one on either side of this bud. In boys, they grow together to form the scrotum, and in girls a slit arises between the swellings and develops into a vagina.

The boy's primitive testicles, like the girl's ovaries, are located deep inside the abdominal cavity. An inspection of the interior of the testicles by means of a microscope clearly reveals the ducts of the testicles, in which the precursors of sperm have already begun to develop. The ovaries already contain large numbers of tiny follicles, each containing an ovum. As early as the fourth fetal month, the five million ova that are produced in a woman's lifetime have already been formed. In the man, on

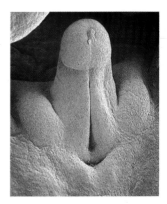

Eight weeks old. The external sex organs of both sexes are still strikingly similar, but the internal sex organs already manifest clear differences.

Seven weeks, 25 mm (about 1 inch).

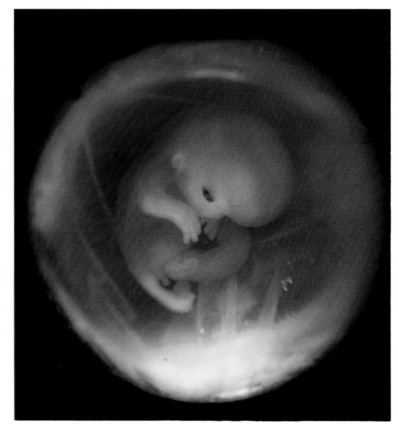

Boy

Near right: the penis of a 16-week-old fetus. *Middle*: the testicles (still in the abdomen) in week 13. *Far right*: cross section of a testicle (16 weeks), showing one of the convoluted seminal vesicles in which sperm are formed. Already, the primitive sperm are in position and the cells colored blue are forming the male sex hormone.

Girl

The female fetus's counterpart to the penis, the clitoris, is visible between the labia in week 21. The next picture shows the ovaries as they are in week 11. A cross section of the budding ovary of a newborn baby girl reveals a primitive ovum cell surrounded by nutrient cells.

the other hand, new sperm capable of fertilizing an ovum, are formed right up to an advanced age.

In the fetal stage, some ovarian follicles already grow to a fairly considerable size under the influence of hormones from the mother's pituitary gland. However, development never proceeds as far as ovulation, and no ova probably reach full maturity, since the mother's hormonal balance is not prepared for ovulation during her pregnancy either.

A pregnant woman who takes hormones, for example to build up her muscles, runs the risk of impairing the development of the fetal sex organs, regardless of whether the fetus is male or female.

If they wish, the parents-to-be can learn the sex of the embryo or fetus long before birth by various fetal-diagnostic methods. Both amniocentesis and chorionic villus sampling (CVS) can provide, by chromosome determination, a 100 percent reliable answer, and—at least in the latter half of pregnancy—an ordinary ultrasound scan usually yields the same information.

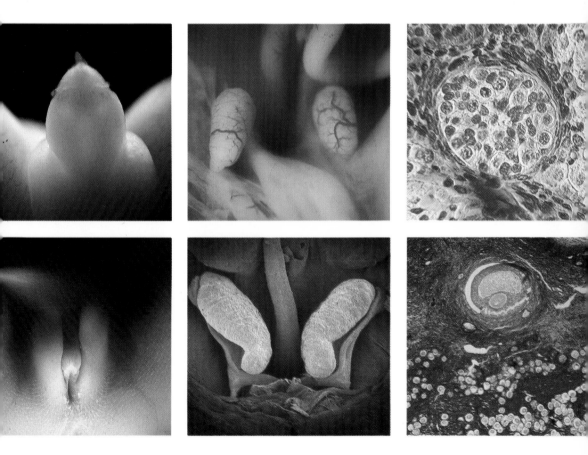

Fetal diagnosis — a visual technique

Although ultrasound technology has made it possible to monitor the fetus repeatedly during its development, there are sometimes reasons for examining the contents of the uterus by means of an instrument called a fetoscope. This is a type of telescope measuring only a few milimeters in diameter, inserted through the abdominal wall close to the navel.

The procedure takes place with the mother under general anesthesia, and considerable skill is required in order not to injure the fetus. Wide-angled optics permit overviews of almost the whole fetus, but the doctor is usually more interested in details, such as a hand, a foot or the genitals.

In the fetus illustrated here, the aim was to check the presence of an unusual bone disorder which cannot be clearly diagnosed by ultrasound. The examination went smoothly, and the baby, *insert*, was entirely healthy at the time of birth 22 weeks later.

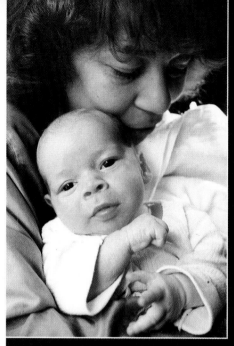

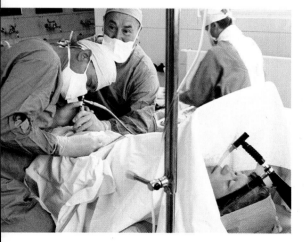

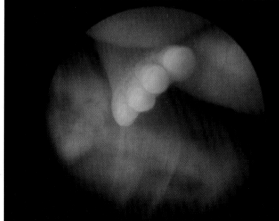

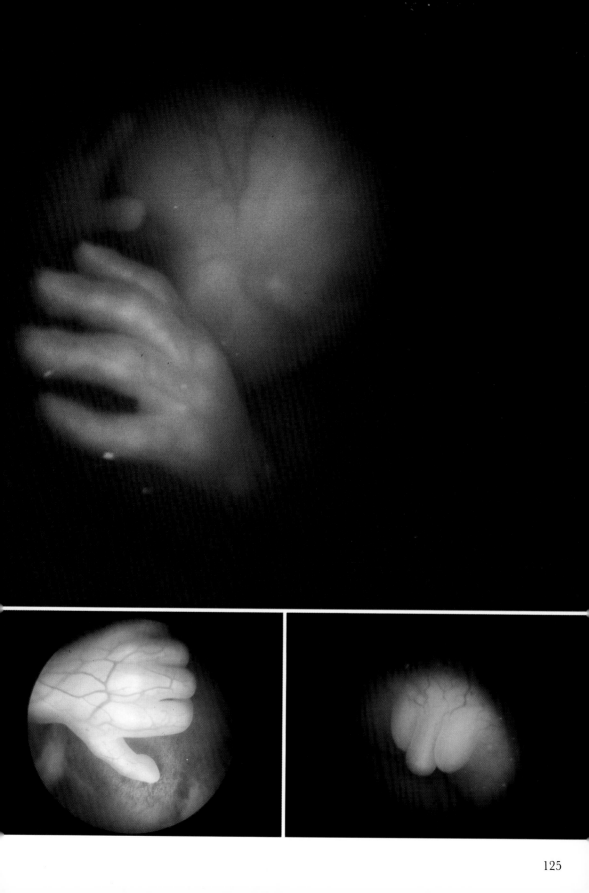

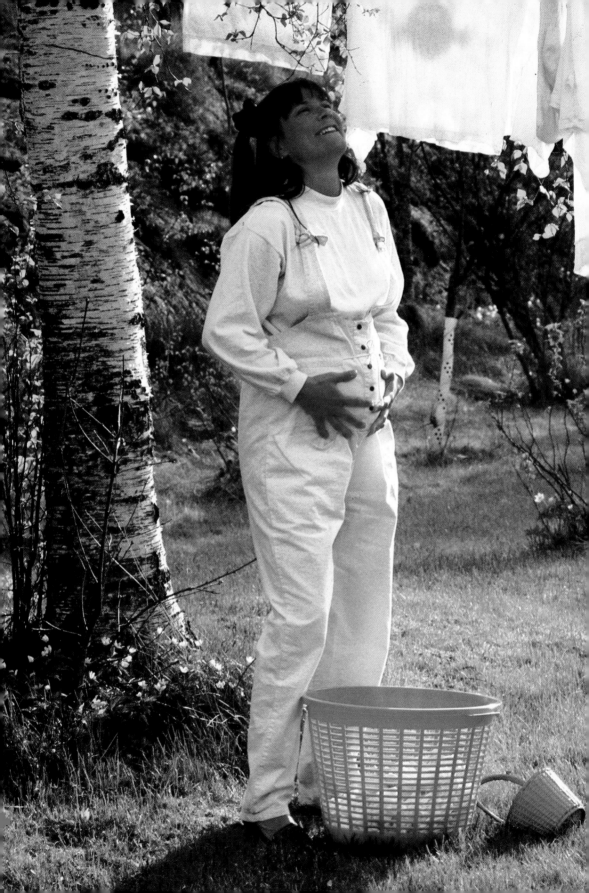

Halfway to Birth

Roughly halfway through pregnancy, i.e. 18 to 20 weeks after the last menstrual period began, a woman begins to notice the first, fluttery fetal movements. If she does not know how they are supposed to feel, it takes her longer to be certain; women who are pregnant for the first time ("primigravida") usually notice the motions a couple of weeks later than those who have previously given birth ("multigravida"). The first signs cannot be taught—they must be experienced. Women liken them to bubbles or butterfly wings or the twitching of a fish's tail.

The woman has by now usually put on several pounds, and her abdomen is beginning to be slightly rounded. The upper portion of the uterus has not reached the level of the navel and there is still ample room. Breathing is unaffected, the nausea has ceased and most women find this the best phase of pregnancy, both mentally and physically. A sensation of warmth—as if the body contained a built-in heater—is common.

Prenatal visits to the doctor or clinic continue, usually once a month, with routine checks of urine, blood pressure and measurements of the uterus. Increased discharge from the vagina is entirely natural, but if this becomes excessive, irritating or malodorous, it should be mentioned to the doctor or midwife. The reason is often a yeast infection that can easily be treated.

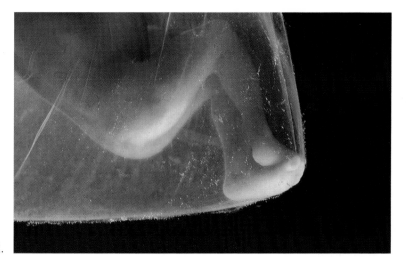

The first kicks are an extraordinary sensation, especially for a woman who has never felt them before. By this time, she is usually in week 18–20 of her pregnancy, but the fetus has already, in fact, been moving inside the uterus for many weeks. Only now, however, do the movements become strong enough to make themselves felt through the abdominal wall.

Common complaints

Varicose veins and hemorrhoids (piles) are common ailments in the third trimester. The reason for both is the same: the enlarged uterus is pressing on large veins in the pelvis. This makes blood pressure in the veins higher than normal and causes the veins to swell. This may lead to damage to the valves located in the veins, causing the blood to pool and the blood vessels to expand even further ("ballooning").

While some valve damage does not heal itself after delivery, it is nevertheless advisable to delay surgical treatment until three or four months after delivery, to see if the varicose veins remain. Avoiding long periods of standing and using support stockings can help. Hemorrhoids seldom need to be operated on and usually heal after delivery, especially if the constipation that can be another cause of these troubles is overcome. A diet full of fruit, vegetables and whole grains, as well as exercise, can help avoid the straining that leads to hemorrhoids.

Another ailment arising, in particular, during the third trimester of pregnancy is leg cramps, which may be due to disturbed blood circulation, pressure on nerves, or salt or calcium deficiences. Massage and keeping the toes from pointing straight down can help. Indigestion and heartburn may also sometimes be troublesome. Smaller, more frequent meals and antacids, which are not considered dangerous to the fetus, can help ease digestion.

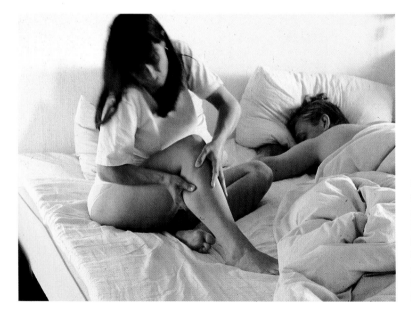

Cramps or aches in the calves are fairly common when the abdomen is beginning to feel heavy and the working day has been long. When the nearest available masseur is asleep, a woman can try walking about, or kneading the muscles herself.

Keeping fit

In many countries a pregnant woman is pampered in such a way that she becomes overly passive. Resting one's way through pregnancy is, in general, inadvisable for both body and spirit. If a woman has a physically active job, that exercise may be enough; but if her job is sedentary, an enjoyable form of physical activity is particularly important in pregnancy. Swimming, tennis, hiking, aerobics— most any favorite sport will do, but contact sports are not appropriate.

Special gymnastic exercises have also been designed for pregnant women. These help to train groups of muscles used during the actual delivery. Local childbirth education groups may offer exercise classes or be able to suggest where to find instruction. The pelvic muscles may be exercised by means of contractions. Pelvic-floor contractions are advisable both before and after birth, in order for the stretched muscles to regain their normal suppleness.

Pregnancy imposes heavy strains on the back, since the expectant mother must counterbalance her expanding and increasingly heavy abdomen. It is also an advantage to have mobile, supple back muscles in the course of labor. Back exercises therefore form a vital part of the prenatal keep-fit program. It is important that any exercise programs for pregnant women be planned by teachers with appropriate experience.

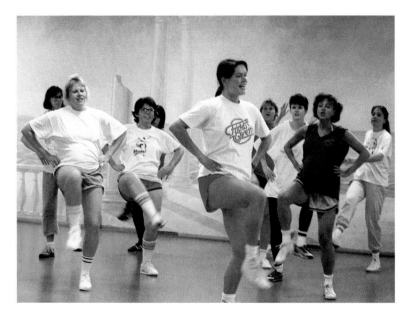

The body is a dynamic construction that does not thrive when staying still. Pregnant women, too, should keep moving about as much as possible. If everyday activities are sedentary, exercise classes for mothers-to-be can be fun and very beneficial if taught by an experienced person.

Preparing mind and body

Not only is it important for the mother to be in good physical condition before delivery; both parents should be mentally well prepared. Clinics and hospitals and independent childbirth education groups therefore offer courses for prospective parents of both sexes. Preparations may include relaxation exercises, and sometimes special breathing instruction as well as baby care. Learning to reduce tension in every muscle of the body, and to lie in a relaxed state—almost at a lower level of consciousness—is a great help during labor. Tension increases the pain experienced during contractions and also the resulting fa-

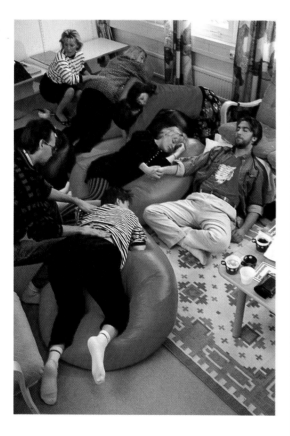

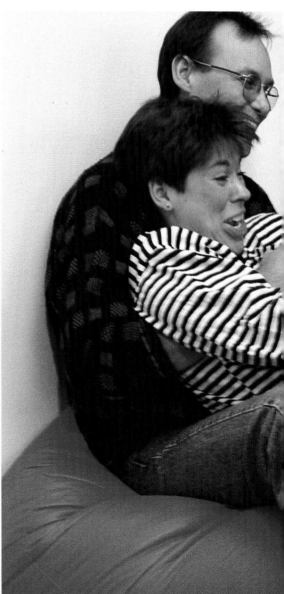

In the second half of pregnancy, it is a good idea to start practicing relaxation, preferably in the company of other expectant parents. Relaxation is a vital element in pain relief, and so is back massage. Here, the father has a chance to lend a hand! In the picture to the right, the group has reached practical exercises in the delivery situation, and dolls can then serve a useful purpose.

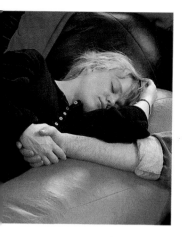

tigue. For this reason, psychological preparation, sometimes known as *psychoprophylaxis* (psyche = mind, prophylaxis = prevention), may be just as important as physical training. Actually, these are inseparable. Learning some anatomy, together with practical and detailed instruction as to what delivery really involves, gives many couples a sense of security when the time comes to give birth. Pregnancy is an opportunity to become more familiar with one's own body and to learn ways to deal with stress and tension that will be valuable long after the birth experience. In choosing a childbirth education class, couples can consult not only with their doctor, clinic, or new parents, but also with any local Lamaze, childbirth education associations or, in the U.K., the National Childbirth Trust.

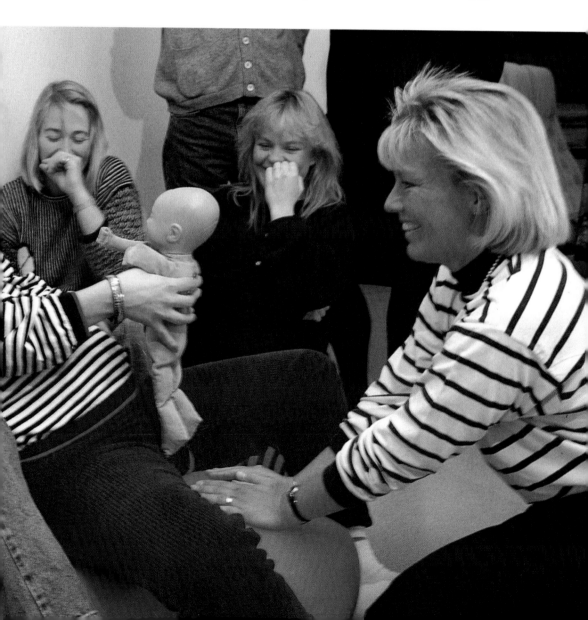

Visiting the hospital

An important part of the preparations, especially for first-time mothers, is a visit to the hospital where the birth will take place. Preferably both parents should do so, in order to learn about the procedure in a delivery room. If this is not offered by hospital or childbirth education classes, parents can ask for it. In addition to showing the room where the birth will take place, someone from the staff can explain all the equipment, the workings of the bed, the monitoring devices available and their purpose, and various methods of alleviating pain, such as nitrous oxide, "gas and air," and injections to numb the nerves. Many women feel an extra sense of security knowing these measures are available, in addition to the relaxation and breathing techniques learned in the childbirth education classes.

Now, pregnancy, delivery and their own future parental role begin to seem real to parents. They both will have many questions and should have no hesitation in asking them. If the woman and her partner have prepared for childbirth together and know, insofar as possible, what to expect, the prospects of the actual delivery being a joyful experience and a happy memory for the future are greatly improved. More and more couples are becoming fully informed and investigating all the options open to them. The expectant father's presence and encouragement is a valuable support, and in many cases he can also provide help and thereby feel himself to be more of a participant.

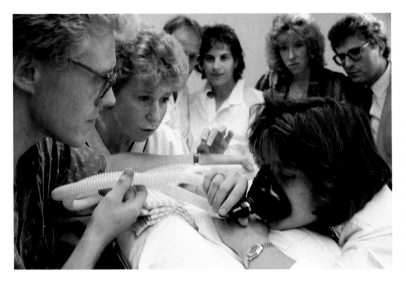

Courses for expectant parents often include group visits to a maternity unit in a hospital. Here, parents-to-be are acquainting themselves with a situation that is looming ever closer. It feels reassuring to have tried out the anesthesia mask and learned how it works in case the need to use it in earnest arises.

Trying out delivery positions

Most women give birth reclining in a semi-sitting position, in a hospital bed. This has not always been the case. The traditional modern delivery position was probably something introduced by doctors in hospitals so that they could more easily handle the delivery and intervene if necessary.

Nowadays, women are often free to choose the position in which they want to give birth. In olden times— and to this day among primitive peoples—women took advantage of the force of gravity, giving birth in a standing, kneeling or hanging position, as shown in the pictures below. Modern versions of these same positions are illustrated alongside.

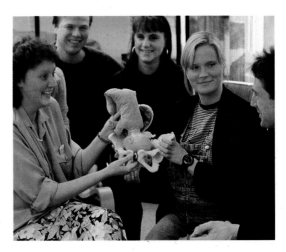

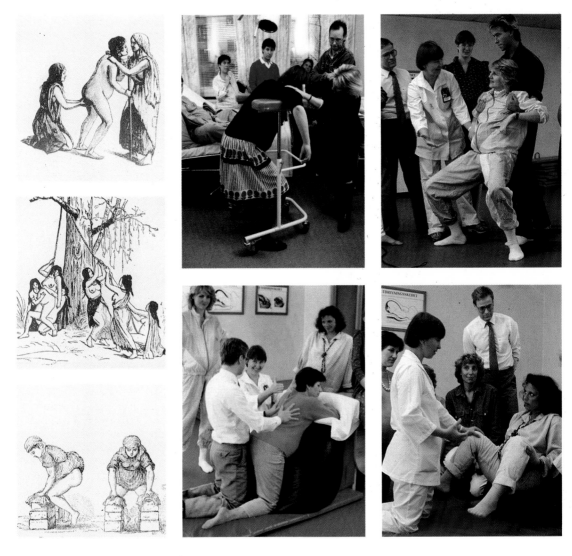

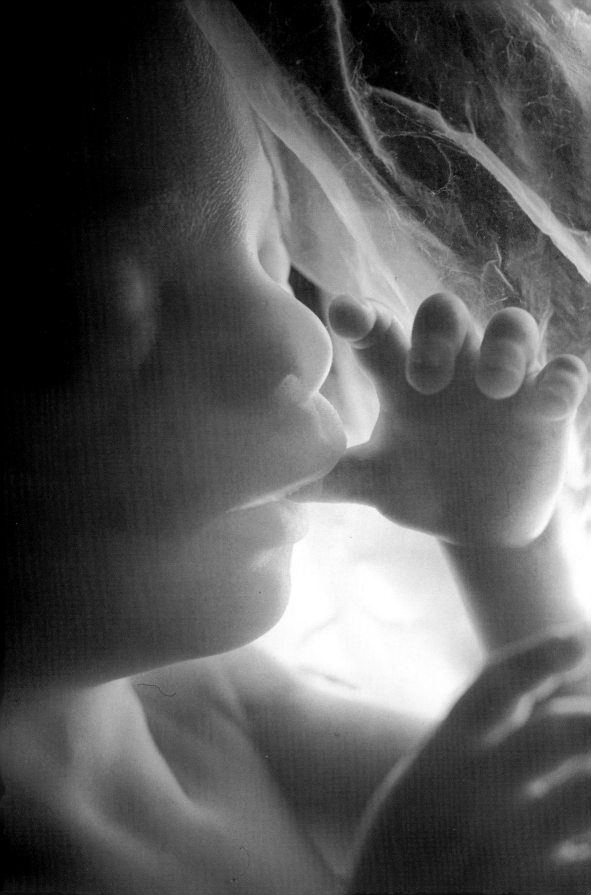

Almost Ready for Life

The fetus lies in a well-protected position, suspended in the amniotic fluid deep inside the uterus. But this does not mean that it is isolated from the outside world. The fetus is surrounded by vibrations and noises, which it can begin to perceive as early as in the fifth month: blood swishing and pounding in the mother's blood vessels, the rumbling of her stomach and intestines, and her voice, which resounds through her body.

Other sounds penetrate from the world outside, and loud noises can make the fetal heart beat faster and perhaps even make the whole fetus tremble. In due course, it learns to recognize certain patterns in the sound environment, and may grasp the difference between its parents' voices. The mother gradually notices that her fetus reacts to what is going on around her, and interprets this as the steady awakening of consciousness.

The fetus lives in a shadowy world, but some light penetrates through the mother's abdominal wall and the wall of the uterus. The eyes are closed until the seventh month, but after that we can be fairly sure that the fetus perceives light as a reddish shimmer.

After 24 weeks of pregnancy, when the fetus weighs roughly half a kilo (a little over 1 pound), it begins to have a chance of survival, though the risk of handicap is still high.

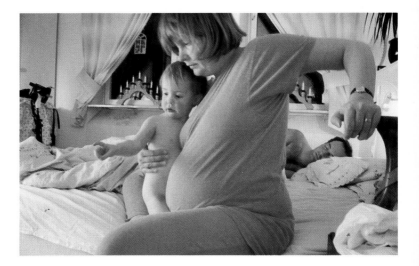

Already, the hand is a tiny, exquisite work of art. In this 4½-month-old fetus, the body's systems are now being tested. It moves and waves its arms. A finger touching its lips precipitates a slight sucking reflex.

Right: a mother-to-be, heavily pregnant and tired, whose daily tasks are not yet done. Big sister-to-be also needs attention.

The fetus puts on weight

During the last two months in the uterus, the fetus builds up a protective layer of fat in its dermis. Its weight increases by roughly 200 grams (almost half a pound) a week. The mother, however, may have to watch her weight. Overeating in pregnancy can be a problem. Not only is the mother affected, but the fetus may start life with an excess supply of fat. A high birth weight is not always a sign that the uterine environment has been optimal. One classic example of this is women with diabetes. If the blood-sugar level has been awry during pregnancy, the fetus will be large and bloated, and not thrive particularly well. Birth weights between four and five kilos (9–12 pounds) in such cases are not uncommon, and this in turn may make the actual delivery more difficult.

Nor is it good for the fetus if the mother eats inadequately

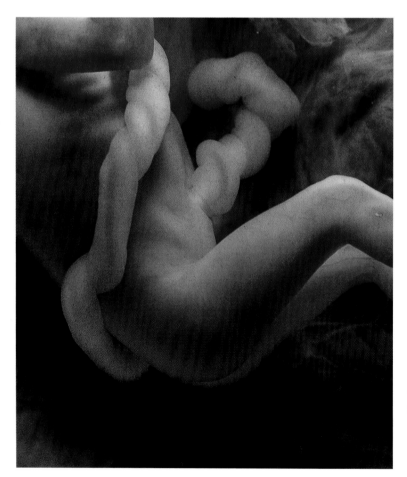

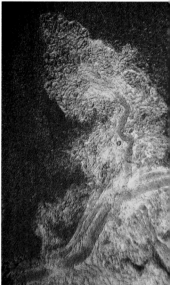

The fetal lifeline, the umbilical cord, is strong and tough and assumes impressive dimensions by the end of pregnancy. The blood vessels are embedded in a firm, gelatinous substance that prevents kinks or knots in the cord that might cut off the blood supply.

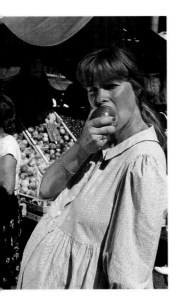

during pregnancy, although it may be said with some truth that the fetus is nourished at the expense of the mother. Malnutrition during pregnancy, especially associated with vitamin and mineral deficiency, is one of the major global problems, since the foundations of a number of brain functions are laid before a baby is born. If the mother and thus the fetus do not receive a balanced diet, brain development may be impaired. At birth, the baby's brain has hundreds of billions of nerve cells formed and developed throughout fetal life, but it is believed that, after birth, no new nerve cells arise. We must therefore take care of our brain cells, both during the fetal stage and as children and adults. Slimming diets during pregnancy are inadvisable. It is also important that the mother should not impair her baby's brain development by smoking, drinking alcohol or taking, for example, large doses of tranquilizers.

The exchange of placental nutrients and oxygen between the maternal and fetal blood takes place in tiny, finger-like projections (the chorionic villi), submerged in tissues filled with maternal blood. *Left*, the picture shows a chorionic villus surrounded by the mother's blood. In each such villus, fetal blood circulates through a minute blood vessel (capillary).

Right, we see the tip of a protrusion from the placenta, greatly magnified, containing the fetal blood cells in the U-shaped capillary. Only a thin membrane separates it from the mother's red blood cells. Through this membrane, oxygen and nutrients are transferred. All the fetal waste products pass back through the membrane. Once the fetal blood cells are replete with oxygen, their color changes to bright red.

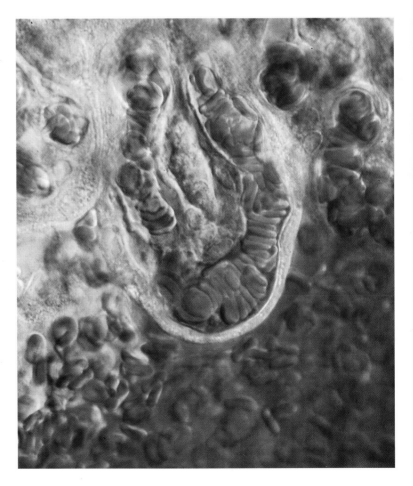

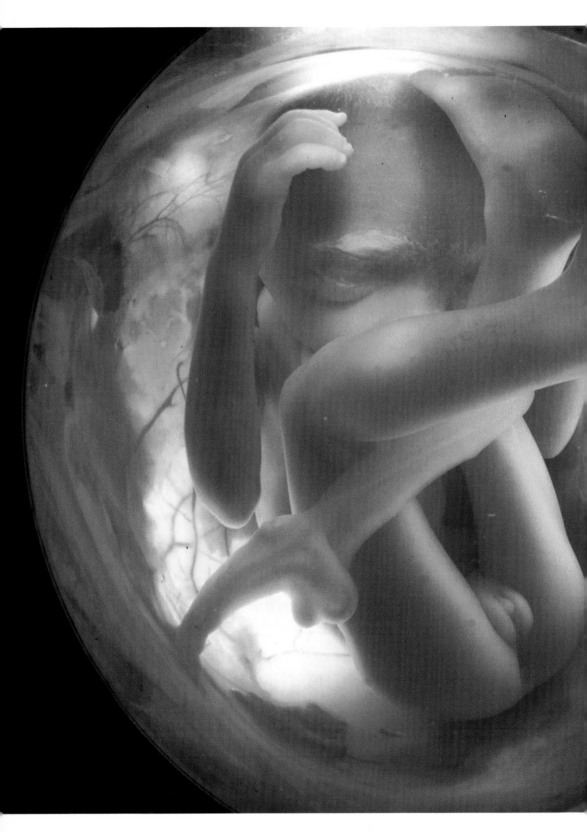

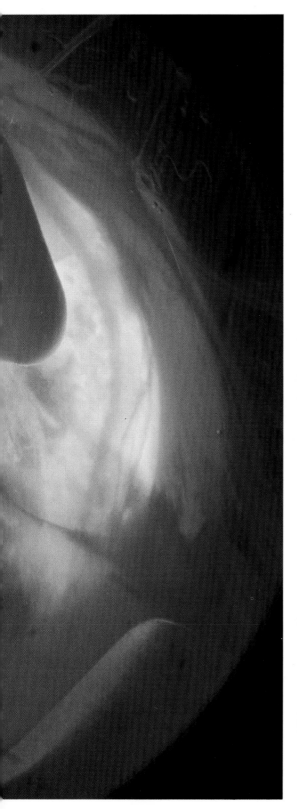

Constant training

A fetus starts moving as early as in the eighth week of pregnancy, and continues until birth. For a long time, the motions consist of primitive reflexes in arms and legs, but in the fifth month, they become more deliberate and coordinated. This is a sign that the nerve fibers are being connected. The fetus stretches, grasps and turns. All these movements are necessary for muscular and skeletal growth, and for the development of fine motor ability. If a woman notices that these fetal movements are perceptibly reduced, or absent, for a day or so she should consult a clinic or doctor for an extra check.

Eighteen weeks, 24 cm (about 9 inches).

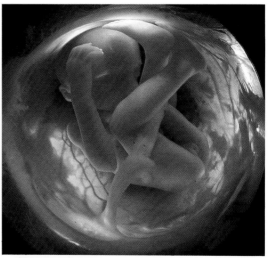

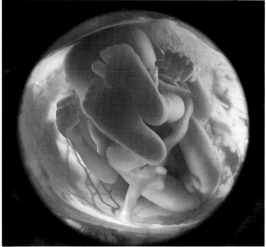

Running out of space

Until the seventh month of pregnancy, the fetus can move freely and even turn a somersault but at about this time, it becomes a squeeze and almost all the available room in the uterus is filled up.

The quantity of amniotic fluid increases at the end of pregnancy, and at the time of delivery there is usually between 0.5 and 1.5 liters (1–3 pints). The amniotic fluid is a sterile solution that is rapidly renewed by means of the fetus's urine secretion. The slight cloudiness is caused by the discarded fetal cells and excess vernix suspended in the fluid, but nutrients and products necessary for lung development and maturation are also present. The fetus swallows the amniotic fluid and gives the alimentary canal practice. Sometimes the fetus may get hiccups, which the mother experiences as small, cramp-like jerks.

Eight months, 45 cm (18 inches).

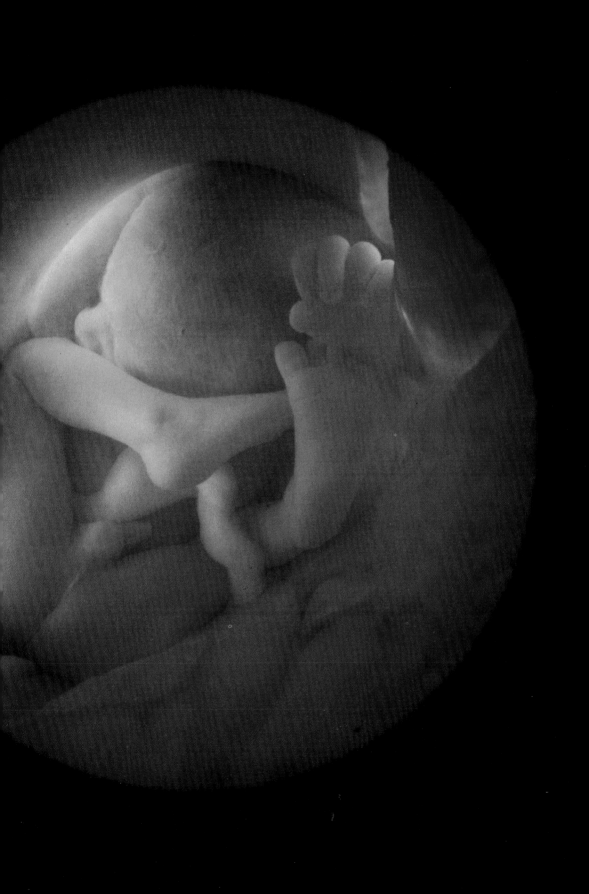

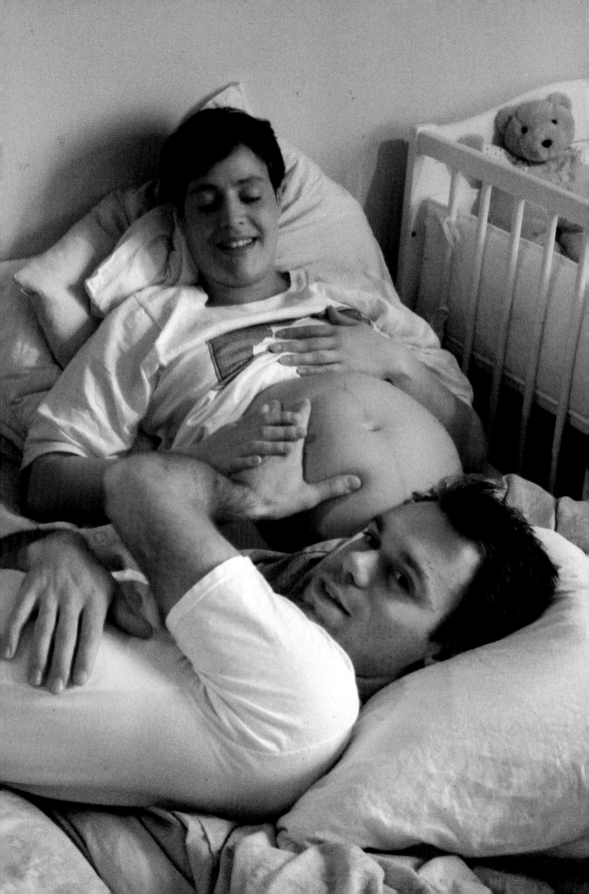

The Last Long Weeks

The abdomen becomes exceedingly large toward the end of pregnancy. Most expectant mothers find its weight troublesome; many suffer from back pain, and their curiosity and longing to see the baby is mixed with anxiety about the actual delivery. Downward pressure on the bladder, which makes it difficult to retain urine, is often experienced as the most troublesome symptom. Others find the upward pressure toward the chest and difficulty in breathing deeply the greatest strain.

In late pregnancy, some women find it hard to sleep at night and may therefore need to rest for an hour or so in the daytime; this benefits the fetus as well. It is important to be rested, as preparation both for delivery and for the psychological adjustment to the maternal role. Many women cut down their hours at work, if they have not already started their leave.

During the last few weeks of pregnancy, numerous small snacks during the day are more digestible than a couple of large meals. This is a period in which the mother can gather energy for the "grand finale." The ideal snacks at this time are fresh fruit and fiber-rich vegetables, and plenty of cottage cheese and yoghurt, preferably with whole-grain cereals, raisins and nuts.

If delivery is slightly delayed, this is seldom anything to worry about—a normal pregnancy varies from 38 to 42 weeks.

By this late stage, the expectant belly is the focus of much interest. All together, the woman's weight usually increases by 10–15 kg (25–35 pounds) during pregnancy. The fetus accounts for about one third of this weight gain, while much of the remainder is accounted for by the placenta, the amniotic fluid, the enlarged uterus and breasts and the greater volume of blood.

Now the waiting is almost over—and the baby's crib is already made up and ready for the new occupant!

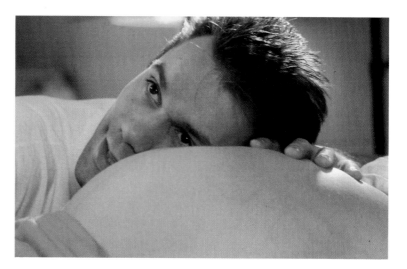

That's my heart you're listening to!

Around four weeks before the expected delivery date, the mother-to-be begins to go to the doctor or clinic more frequently to be weighed, have her blood pressure taken and hand in a urine sample. The doctor, nurse or midwife also measures the growth of her abdomen and enters the figures on a graph showing a normal projection of the baby's growth. He or she also checks the position of the fetus—head downward, as in 97 percent of cases, or otherwise? An amplifier enables the mother and future brothers or sisters to hear the beat of the fetal heart. It seems to say: "This is me—that's my heart you're listening to!"

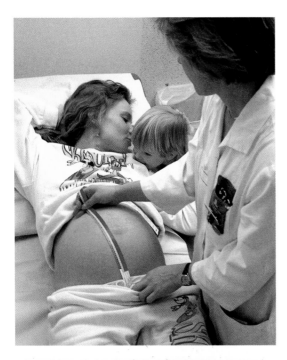

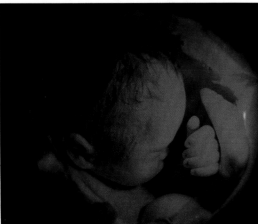

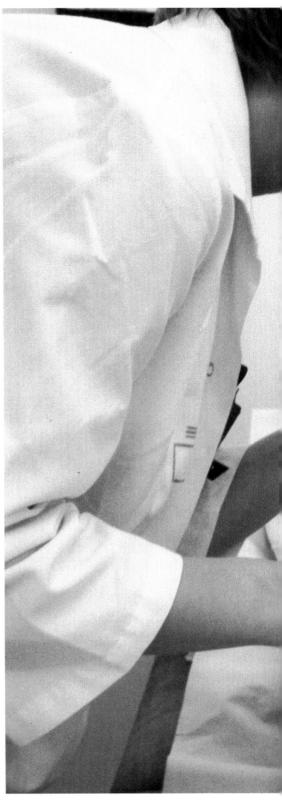

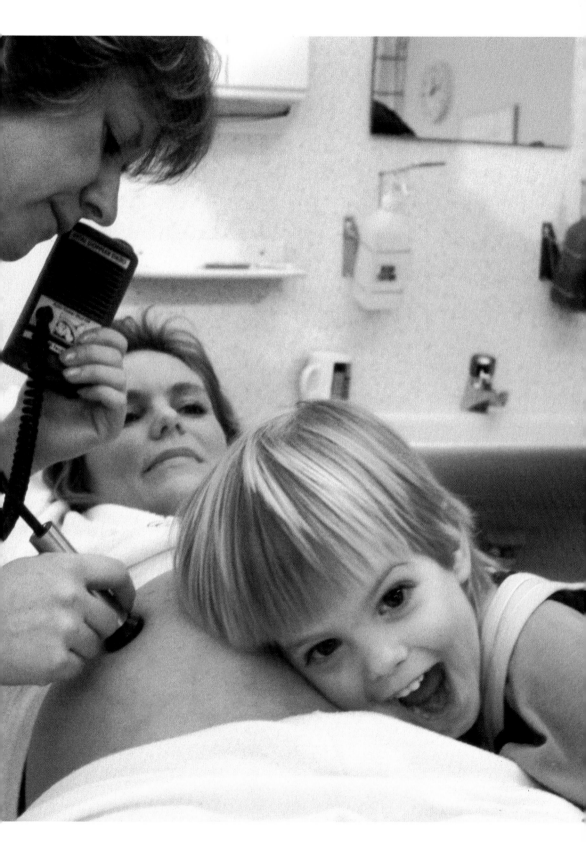

Position of the fetus

In order to plan the delivery, the doctor and midwife must make careful assessments of the fetus's position in the uterus. In the great majority of cases (97 percent), the head lies downward (cephalic presentation); delivery is then easiest. After the 35th week, a fetus seldom rotates spontaneously, so one must either content oneself with the presentation or try to adjust it. If the baby feels very large and the mother is small, tests may be done to determine whether her pelvic measurements are sufficient for the baby to pass. If the baby is delivered legs or bottom first (breech presentation), even larger pelvic dimensions are required for a vaginal birth to take place successfully.

The doctor can also try to turn the baby. This is known as external cephalic version (ECV), and is a maneuver that requires experience and should always be carried out by an obstetrician at a hospital, where there are facilities to deal with any complications that may arise.

Some obstetricians prefer to deliver babies in breech positions by means of *cesarean sections*, since they consider this less of a risk for the baby. Others prefer to attempt the natural way, but with the option of an emergency cesarean if labor becomes too difficult, or if the baby suddenly shows signs of distress. Babies lying in a transverse position, i.e. across the uterus, are also often born by cesarean section. If there is more than one baby in the uterus (twins or triplets), each baby is usually so small that natural childbirth seldom poses any problems.

The number of babies delivered by cesarean section has increased for various reasons. The main one is undoubtedly that abdominal surgery is less hazardous than it used to be; the risk of life-threatening infections has diminished sharply owing to more sterile conditions and access to effective antibiotics. There is, however, much concern about cesareans becoming too frequent, i.e. of the method being used unnecessarily. At some hospitals in the U.S., more than 30 percent of all babies are delivered in this manner. A certain number of these may be done because of obstetricians' fear of being sued for malpractice.

The basis of all modern obstetric care is a balance between the mother's interest in a delivery that is as natural and comfortable as possible and an endeavor to minimize those risks to the baby's health that are connected with birth. Today, most women can look forward to giving birth as a powerful and exhilarating experience matched by no other in life.

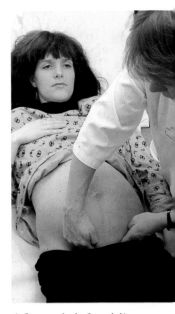

A few weeks before delivery, the fetus settles into one position: usually, the head descends into the birth canal ("engagement"). If the position of the fetus or the placenta will make vaginal delivery too dangerous, a cesarean section may be the best method of delivery.

Future fetal monitoring

To make delivery safer for both mother and baby, one must know exactly how the fetus is lying. Here, the new technique of nuclear magnetic resonance (NMR) is an invincible rival to X rays, especially since it is less hazardous to the fetus. The technique provides images in sharp focus, beautiful and informative (*below right*). Unfortunately, the method is extremely expensive at present—it remains a technique of the future.

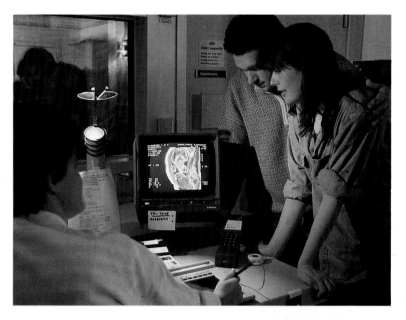

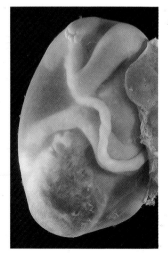

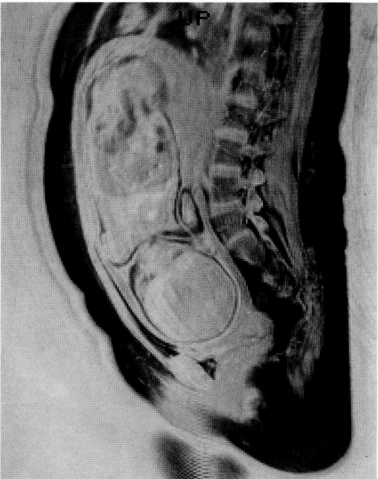

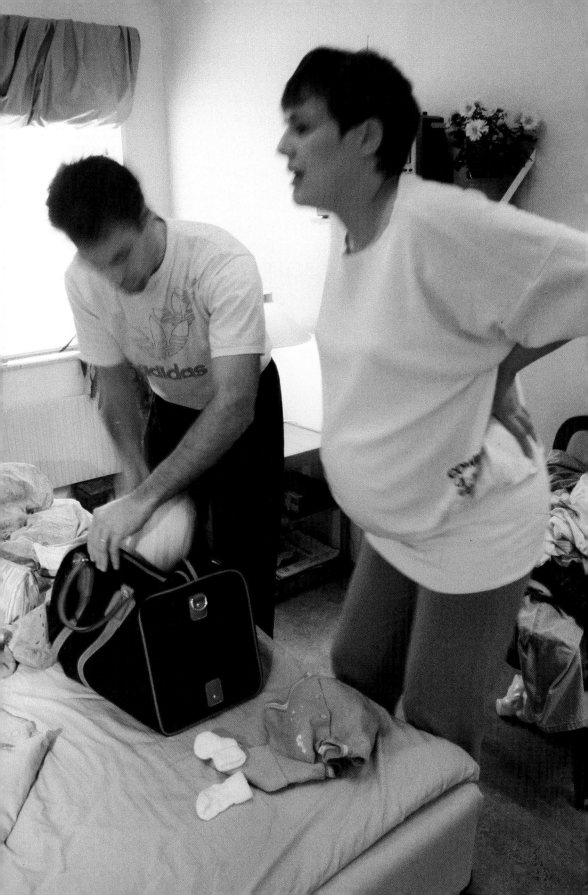

Labor and Delivery

Every pregnant woman should be familiar with three definite signs that delivery is imminent: regular contractions, ruptured membranes ("waters breaking") and a "show" of mucus sometimes mixed with blood.

Uterine contractions are felt by most women at odd times throughout the last weeks of pregnancy. These isolated contractions cause the uterus to become as hard as a ball for one or more minutes. As delivery approaches, these contractions become strong and increasingly regular.

Contractions at intervals of less than ten minutes are a fairly reliable indication that labor has begun. These contractions have been called "labor pains" since time immemorial, since they are—at a later stage, though generally not initially— associated with pain. If the woman is upright, she stops and braces herself during the contractions, perhaps leaning against a chair or a wall. When the contractions are occurring about every five minutes, it is normally time for admission to the hospital. If the woman feels unsure, the best course of action is to call the doctor or midwife.

Labor sometimes begins with amniotic fluid gushing, or starting to flow out of the vagina. This is a sign that the amniotic sac ("bag of waters") has ruptured and the mother should always contact the doctor or hospital right away, since there is some risk of complications. In other cases, the sac ruptures during labor.

Before labor starts or in the first stage, the plug of mucus in the cervix loosens and passes out of the vagina. This plug is often slightly mixed with blood and may have loosened in conjunction with negligible contractions that the woman has not even felt.

Physical exertion or pressure on the cervix during sexual intercourse may cause bleeding on a very small scale. This is generally not of concern. However, if at any time the bleeding is heavy, one should of course go straight to the hospital.

Now there is no time to lose. The contractions are coming at five-minute intervals and the ache goes right through to the back. It is time to go to the hospital. Is the suitcase packed and ready?

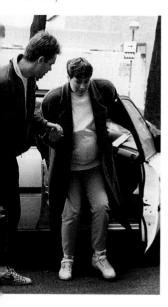

In the hospital

The maternity unit in the hospital is a world in itself—one that the woman has, perhaps, seen on a previous occasion, but only as a spectator. Now, she is suddenly playing the leading role in a drama that is played out nonstop, round the clock, on weekdays and weekends, and is always filled with joy, pain, relief, attended by a company of doctors and nurses and in some cases midwives and other professional staff.

The props on this stage have changed greatly over the past few decades. A visiting grandmother may find the apparatus and monitoring equipment alarming, but on the other hand, the setting has also become more friendly and cheerful, with more comfortable beds, or birth chairs or stools instead of beds in some cases. Today, women have greater freedom to decide how they will give birth; they can walk and move about more freely; they may have relatives or friends with them, perhaps in special cozy private rooms; and they can obtain more, and more effective, help against the pain associated with delivery.

Labor is usually divided into three different stages. The *dilatation stage* begins when the contractions start or the membranes rupture. The cervix gradually opens, until it is "fully dilated" at about 10 cm (just under 4 inches). At the same time, the baby's head (or bottom) pushes and rotates downward to the pelvis. This stage is the longest in labor and takes somewhere from about 6 to 20 hours, less when women have given birth before. These are only averages and it is important to remember that normal labors vary considerably.

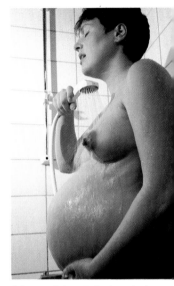

After arriving at the hospital, a hot shower to relax the tension feels good.

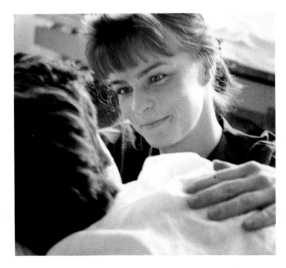

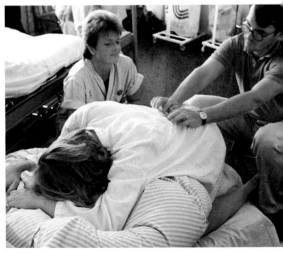

How does it feel? A nurse or midwife looks after the mother-to-be from the start, soothes her and builds up her confidence. The father is also an important person during delivery. He can do a great deal to relieve the pain, for example by massaging the woman's aching back.

The second stage—*the expulsion stage*—lasts from the time the cervix is fully dilated and the baby's head becomes engaged in the pelvis until the baby is born. It is an active stage for the mother, and it is now that she "bears down," pushing out the baby. This stage normally varies from a few minutes to just over an hour. The third stage, the *delivery of the placenta*, begins when the baby is born and continues until the placenta has been expelled. This normally takes about fifteen minutes, but it may take up to an hour or longer. It is usually very easy.

Being born entails considerable stress for the baby. During each contraction, when the placenta and umbilical cord are compressed as the uterine muscles draw together, the supply of oxygen to the baby is curtailed. Initially, the baby's pulse slows down during every strong contraction, but it regains its original rate during the intervals. The baby has a tremendous capacity for withstanding strains, and here the adrenal glands play an important part. These glands secrete large quantities of adrenaline and noradrenaline—hormones that are important in protecting the fetus in the event of an oxygen deficiency, since they promote the heart's pumping capacity, speed up the heart rate, channel blood to the sensitive brain and raise the blood-sugar level. Never again in later life are such large amounts of these stress hormones secreted, and this indicates how stressful it is to be born, but also how well-prepared the baby is for this stress. The hormones are also important in preparing the lungs for life outside the uterus. In particular, adrenaline reduces the formation of liquid in the lungs that has taken place throughout the life of the fetus, and expands the respiratory tract.

The fetus, too, has started to prepare for the imminent event. Its heart beats almost twice as fast as the mother's, and reacts immediately to stress and strain. During delivery, the fetal heartbeat is usually monitored continuously and registered on a strip of paper (CTG). A wooden listening device—an old-fashioned, tried and tested implement—may also be useful, especially at the beginning of labor.

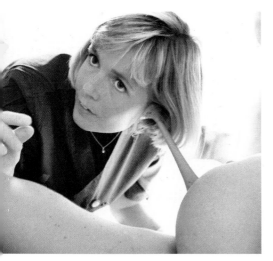

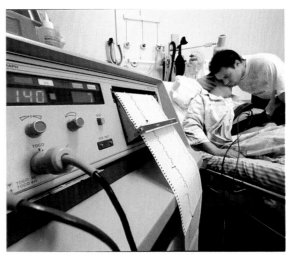

Pain relief

The knowledge acquired and the relaxation technique practiced during pregnancy now play an important part in pain relief. Trying out the various birth positions, experiencing trust, and feeling well looked after markedly reduce the need for conventional pain relief.

The presence of the father-to-be during labor enhances a woman's sense of security. He can help her in various ways, and usually enhances her capacity to withstand pain. The presence of another woman experienced in childbirth, known in some countries as a *doula*, has also been shown to ease pain and shorten labor. It is also worth remembering that pain in conjunction with labor is entirely normal and in no way a dangerous sign. Nor is pain constant; rather, it is associated with the contractions, and this enables the woman to rest in between. In these intervals, she can calm her emotions and collect herself for the next step. Emotionally, it means that she can control her own situation. The body also produces its own pain-relieving hormones—endorphins, as they are called—which dull the perception of pain.

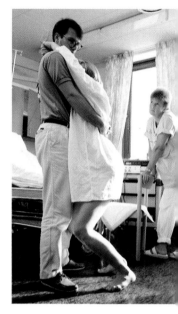

Sometimes it feels good to hang over some strong shoulders and stretch the back muscles. Relaxation is important to relieve the pain of the first stage of labor.

If the woman feels a need for pain relief, there are several different options. One way of relieving pain is an injection of a narcotic analgesic, for example, pethidine. This may lessen pain but may make the woman sleepy or nauseous. It is usually not given within several hours of delivery as it affects the baby. Inhaling *nitrous oxide* mixed with oxygen ("gas and air") through a mask placed on the nose and mouth, is a classic method of alleviating pain. The woman pulls the mask over her mouth when she feels a contraction coming, and she can regulate the quantity inhaled during each contraction. In the intervals, she naturally breathes in the normal way. The disadvantage of this form of pain relief is that it may make the woman sleepy or sick.

Local anesthesia of the nerves surrounding the cervix, or *paracervical block*, as it is called, can provide effective pain relief during the dilatation phase, and the anesthetic itself may also sometimes hasten the cervical dilatation. However, there is some risk of the baby being affected by the anesthetic, and careful monitoring of the baby's cardiac activity, preferably by means of a scalp electrode and a CTG device, is therefore necessary. A local anesthetic in the pelvis—*pudendal block*—is sometimes used in the final stage of delivery. It is administered immediately before the expulsion of the baby. The pudendal nerve runs close to the seat bone (ischium) and is easy to find with the tip of the needle; once the anesthetic has been given, pain in the perineum (pelvic floor) diminishes.

The most effective form of pain relief during birth is provided by an *epidural anesthetic*, which numbs the nerves just as they exit the spinal canal, or a *spinal anesthetic*, which is introduced directly into the spinal canal. This type of nerve block is administered by anesthetists only, since there is a risk of the anesthetic becoming too strong and, as a result, affecting the mother's blood pressure and even her breathing. This, in turn, may have an adverse effect on the baby. Since not only the pain nerves, but also the motor nerves, are blocked by this anesthetic, the mother has difficulty in using her abdominal and pelvic muscles to bear down, with the result that an instrument—a vacuum extractor or forceps—is sometimes needed to help the baby out. The vacuum extractor adheres by means of suction to the baby's head without causing any injury, although the baby generally has a small mark ("caput") for a day or two.

In recent years, throughout the world, there has been a clear tendency away from methods of pain relief which affect the baby or interfere with delivery. Nowadays, there are several *alternative methods of pain relief* that have no adverse effects on either mother or baby. Injecting beads of liquid beneath the skin or transmitting small electric currents through it (TENS = transcutaneous electric nerve stimulation) can enhance the body's own endorphin system in an effective and harmless manner. Acupuncture and hypnosis are other means of relieving pain offered at certain hospitals.

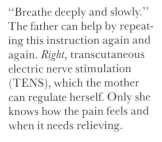

"Breathe deeply and slowly." The father can help by repeating this instruction again and again. *Right*, transcutaneous electric nerve stimulation (TENS), which the mother can regulate herself. Only she knows how the pain feels and when it needs relieving.

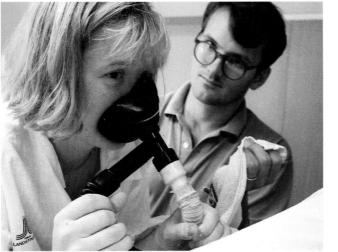

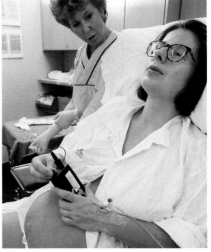

At last, time to push!

Now the contractions are coming regularly: the finale is approaching. Here a midwife is checking how much the cervix has dilated. "Breathe calmly," she says, rest between contractions—Will it never end? Pressure in the genital region is beginning to make itself felt. "Try to push now, push once more—I can already see the hair and glimpse the head. It'll soon be over."

The baby is having a hard time too. There is a surge in production of adrenaline and noradrenaline, the stress hormones, to levels higher than at any time in later life.

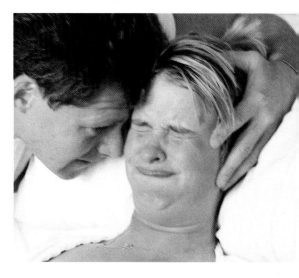

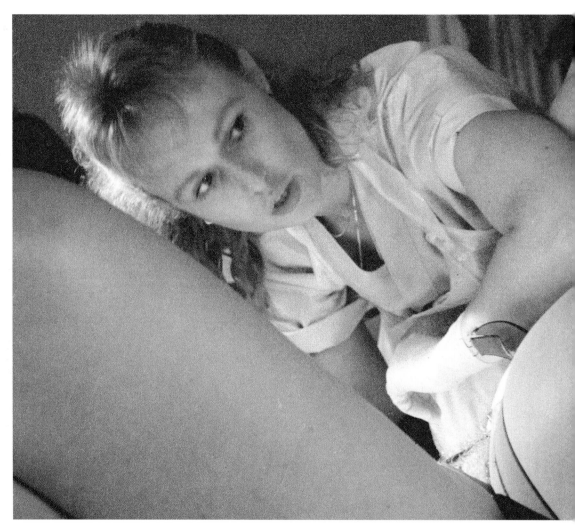

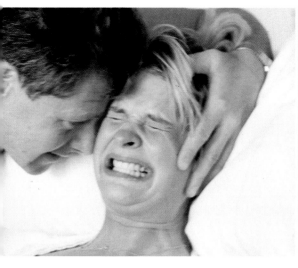

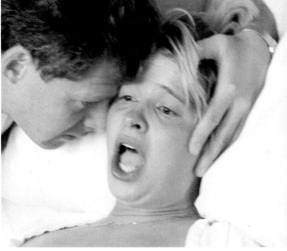

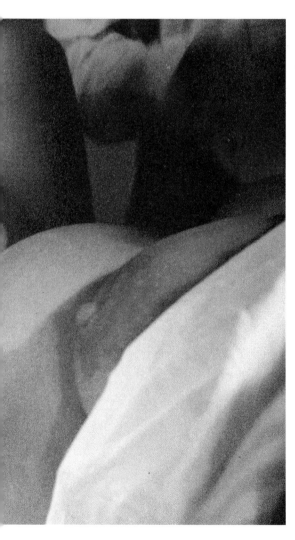

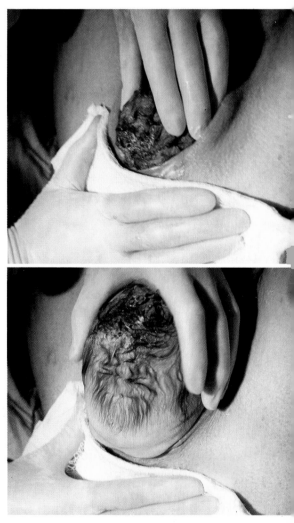

Birth

Now pain, joy, excitement are mingled. The experience of pain varies from one woman to another, depending on sensitivity, expectations and anesthetic effects.

For the baby, birth itself is a cataclysmic event. The adrenaline shock counteracts the oxygen deficiency in the final stage, and prepares the baby for the sudden switch to breathing through the lungs.

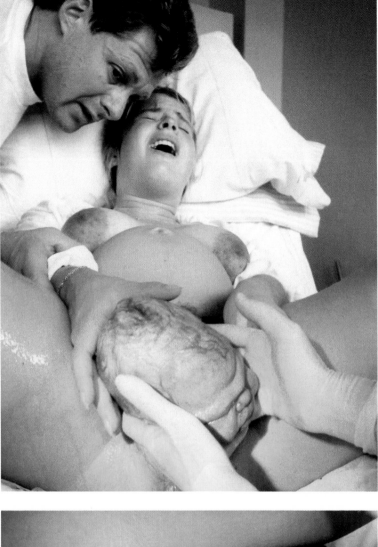

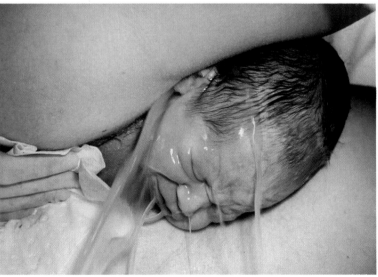

Most of the amniotic fluid escaped earlier. The remainder may be shed during delivery.

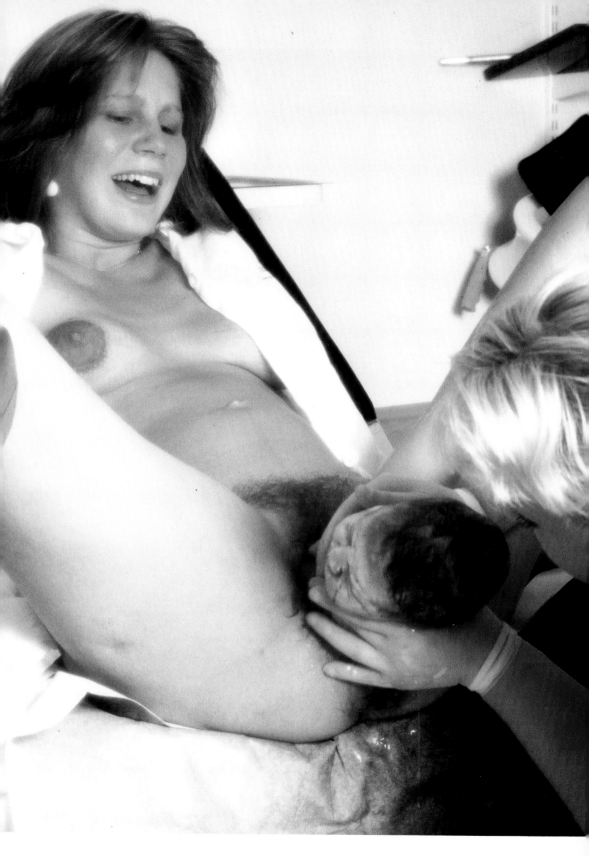

First breath

At last, out in the real world—
a world of dazzling light, cold
air and loud noises. Almost
immediately comes the first
cry—a rare, sometimes
hesitating, sound.

Now 25 million little air
sacs (alveoli) must be filled
with air. Up to now, they have
held fluid, but this is rapidly
expelled in blood and lymph.
The first breaths are among
the most arduous of one's
whole life.

The bloodstream must now
be redirected. The hole in the
partition between the heart's
atria is sealed. Up to now,
oxygen has come from the
mother via the umbilical cord,
but now the baby is self-suffi-
cient: the blood must be di-
rected into the lungs and then
all over the body.

For the parents, this is a
miraculous moment. Such a
tiny human being, so full of
life—their very own child!

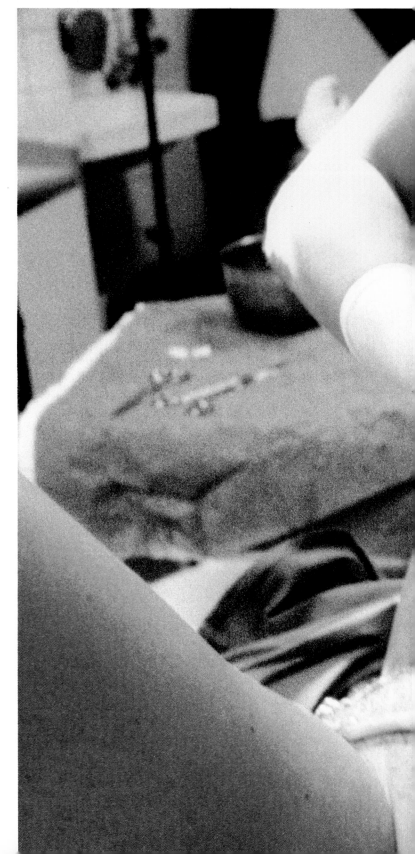

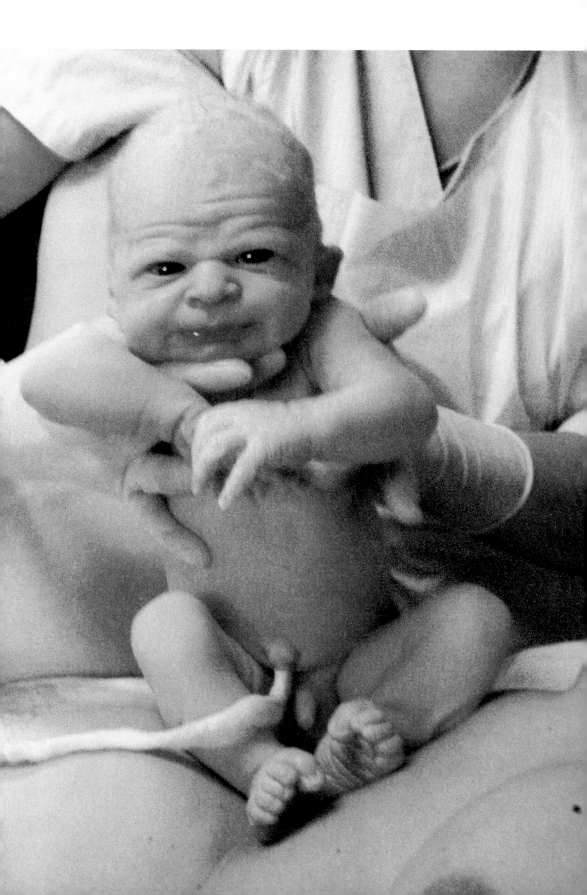

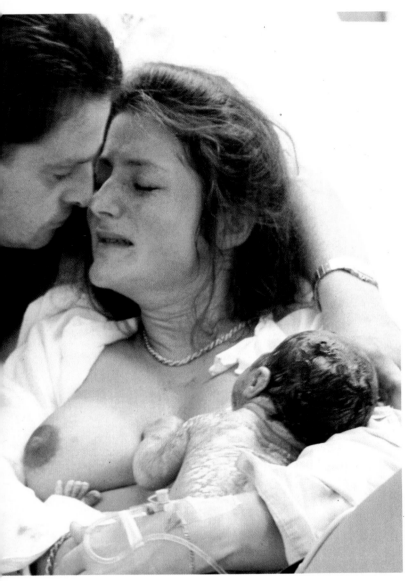

Encounter with the outside world

Look what a beauty I am! Barely a minute old, dazzled by the light, smeared with vernix caseosa, the protective skin grease, the newborn is fully occupied with getting air into his lungs.

The newborn seems relieved to lie on his mother's stomach for a while and relax after all that commotion.

What goes on in the mind of a newborn baby? Suddenly, everything is different. Gone is the cozy life in the amniotic sac: light, sound and smells now assail the sense organs. The baby peers cautiously at his surroundings, first with one eye and then with both. Curiosity is inborn!

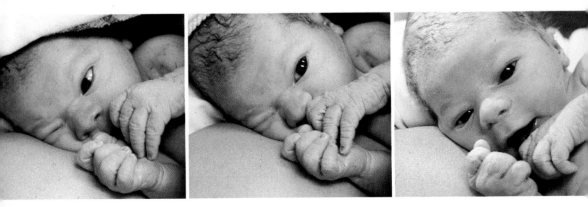

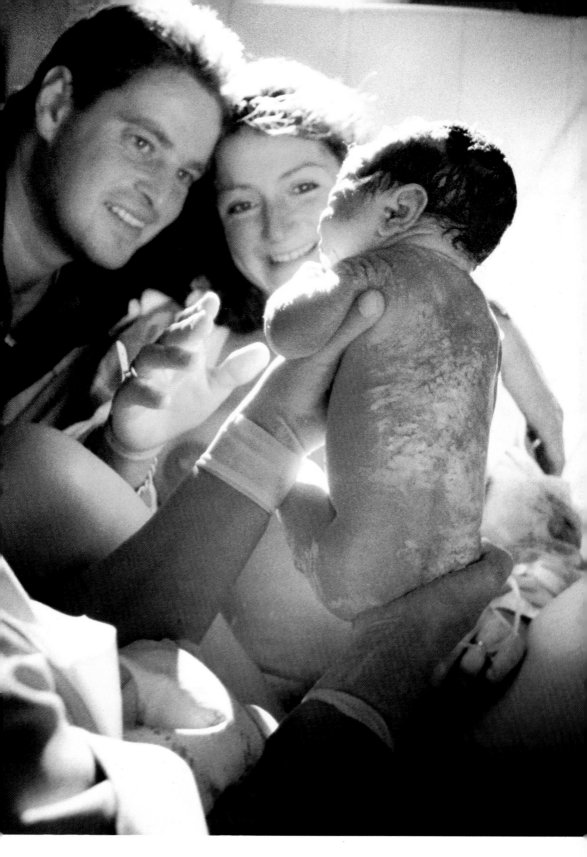

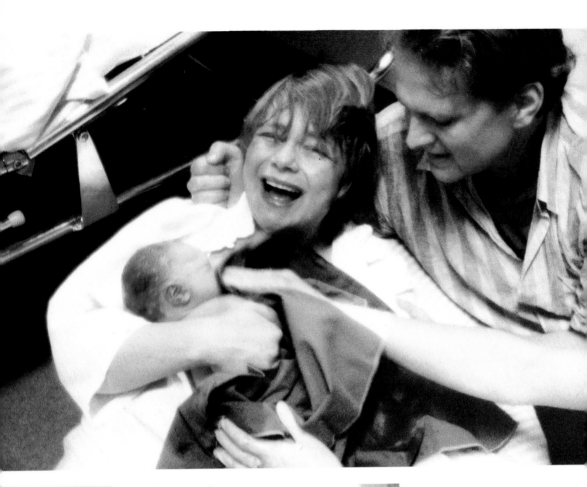

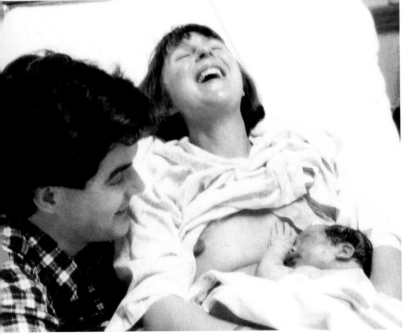

Euphoria

Can it be true? It's all over—
the baby has arrived!

After weeks of waiting,
perhaps with some apprehen-
sion, the parents can finally
stroke and hug the new family
member.

The new family is a small
island of joy amidst the bustle
of the hospital.

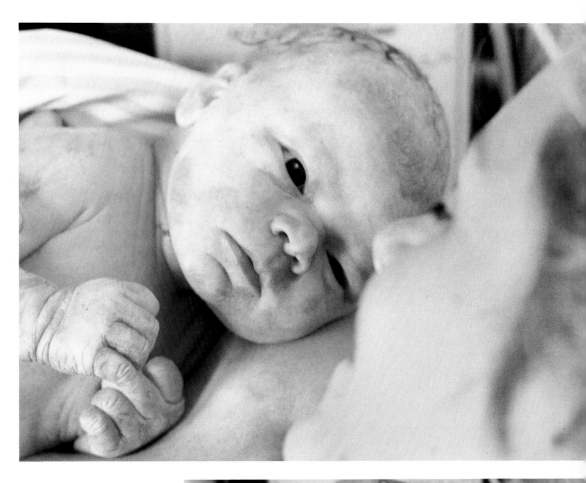

First eye contact

A slightly quizzical look, after all the hullabaloo of the past few hours.

This is a rapturous moment. Mother and baby have struggled together, and now it is time to relax and just enjoy each other, to whisper a few words of tenderness.

This newborn is 4 minutes old.

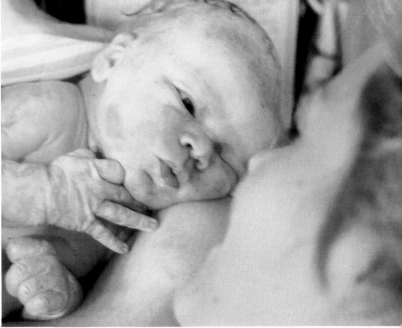

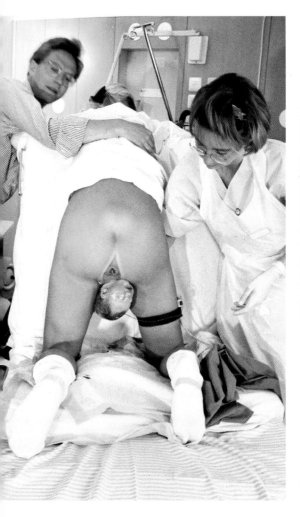

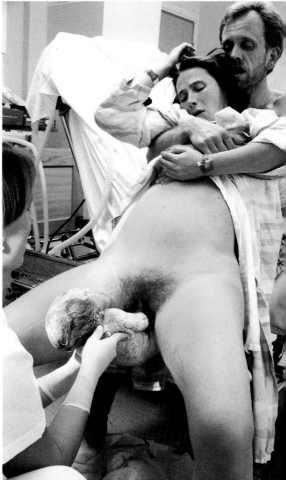

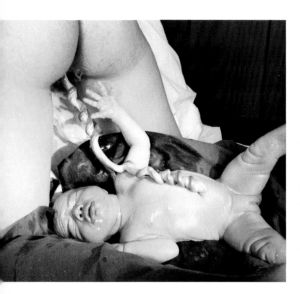

Gravity helps

Giving birth upright or kneeling—the variants are many in present-day delivery rooms. In recent years, women have been allowed ever more freedom to give birth in the position they prefer. Not long ago, it was the rule for women to lie supine in bed: that was the doctor's or midwife's choice. Today, the woman in labor is no longer regarded solely as an amateur in need of constant guidance; the process of delivery follows her needs and inclinations.

These other positions are of course not new. They go back to our ancestors' and to primitive peoples' methods. The woman in labor derives help from the force of gravity. At the same time, if complications arise, it can be life-saving to have specialists and modern equipment within reach.

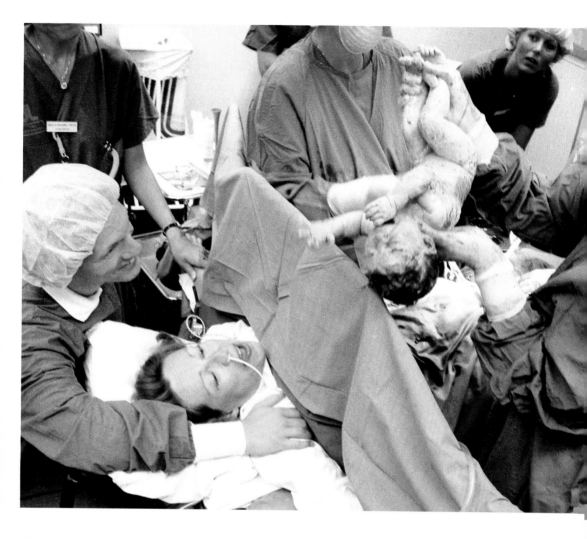

Cesarean section

Cesarean sections are done when the fetus is too large to pass through a narrow pelvis, or if the placenta is located in front of the fetus, among other reasons.

After a spinal or epidural anesthesia, which eliminates sensations of pain in the lower half of the body, the surgeon makes an incision through the abdominal wall and opens the uterus. The amniotic fluid sprays forth, the baby is lifted out and, when the umbilical cord has been cut, placed alongside the mother. In cesarean sections, removing the baby takes only a few minutes.

Nowadays, the father is allowed to attend the operation. The operative site can be screened off so that neither he nor the mother need to see the surgery being performed. Thus, even when a cesarean section is carried out, both parents can establish immediate initial contact with their baby.

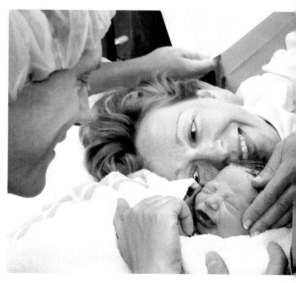

After birth

The umbilical cord is cut immediately after birth, although the placenta remains in the uterus, where it gradually begins to come loose. In the third and final stage of labor, the mother must bear down for the last time, and the placenta is expelled. The uterus can now contract, gradually returning to its original size. The doctor or midwife massages the woman's abdomen gently to facilitate this process. Afterward, the placenta and the fetal membranes must be checked to make sure that they have emerged entirely. Residual fragments of the placenta may give rise to protracted bleeding, and also make it difficult for the uterus to contract.

The doctor or midwife then checks to see if there is any tearing in the vagina and the perineum. If so, the tear is sewn up under local anesthetic. Such tears usually heal very rapidly. The mother is then cleaned up and made comfortable.

When delivery is completed the parents can relax, get to know their baby and be ready for the newborn baby's first meal. Within an hour, the baby usually signals its hunger by a rooting reflex, showing that it is seeking the breast.

In a room empty of apparatus and instruments, calm returns. Soon, a cup of tea or coffee and a freshly made sandwich will be most welcome.

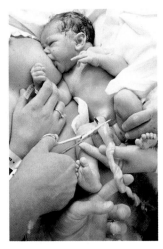

While Dad severs what has been the vital supply line, but now no longer serves any purpose, the baby makes its first attempt to suck at the breast.

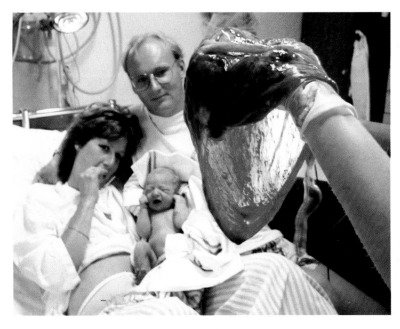

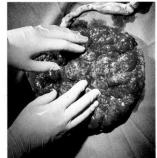

The parents can now see the baby's first home — the amniotic sac with the placenta and umbilical cord.

Above, the whole afterbirth — placenta, cord and membranes — is checked to make sure that nothing has been left behind.

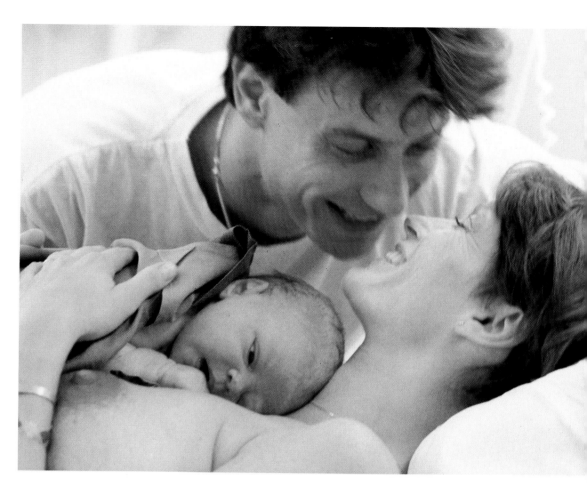

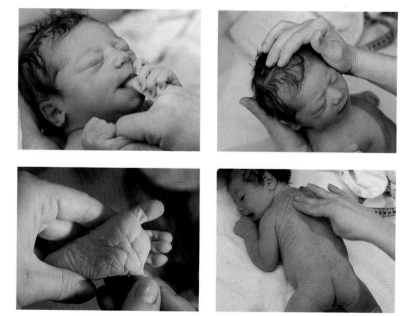

Now, it is time to check over the newborn. Fingers and toes are counted, throat and skull bones and backbone are carefully examined.

Already copying Dad

Newborn babies' ability to imitate their parents' facial expressions is, amazingly enough, evident immediately after birth. Considerably later, infants will start trying to copy the sounds made by their parents. As early as the sixth month, however, experiments have shown that the fetus already has a certain ability to recognize its mother's voice.

The pattern in a newborn baby's manner of imitation is almost invariable, and may be studied for perhaps half an hour after birth, when the baby is quietly alert and wide-awake owing to the surplus of stress hormones produced during delivery. First of all, the baby hears a voice; then it turns to the parent's face and, with great intensity, tries to follow the speech and facial expression. The baby's impressions are gradually linked together, forming an overall experience. After a while, the baby turns away, signaling a desire to break off contact. At this very moment, the first imitation takes place: a yawn, a frown, a tongue sticking out.

Newborns can see best at a distance of 8 to 10 inches, just about the distance at which they see their mothers' faces while feeding. Objects closer or farther away go out of focus.

Up to the age of 3 months, the baby concentrates on imitating facial movements such as opening and closing the mouth, pouting, sticking out the tongue, blinking and so on. In the third month, the baby starts increasingly to imitate speech sounds, and in the fourth month, the more deliberate hand movements begin. Newborn babies have also been observed to move their bodies in synchrony with adult speech. This pattern of development is, of course, full of variations and individual differences.

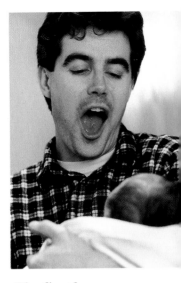

The first lesson

Dad does his best to attract attention. At last eye contact is achieved. What a strange expression. I can do it too!

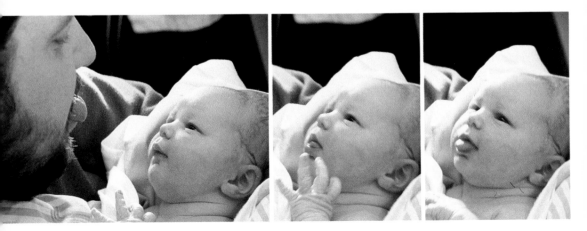

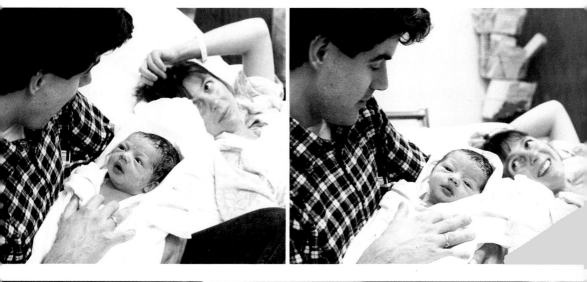

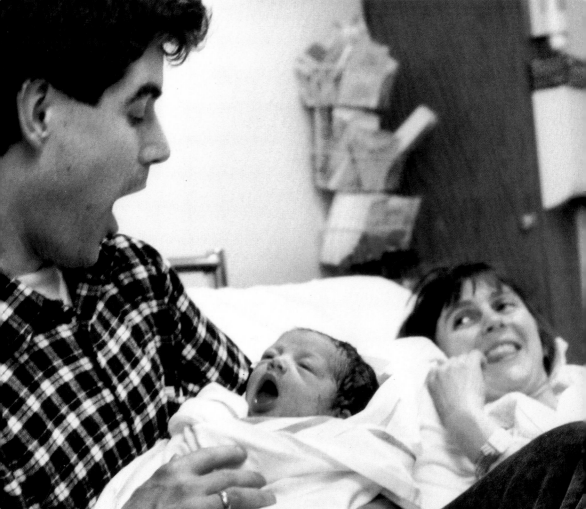

Breastfeeding

Immediately after birth—or within a few hours, at any rate—the baby is put to the mother's breast to learn to suck. The baby's sucking is also necessary in order to set off milk production. A nerve reflex from the nipples reaches certain centers in the lower portion of the brain, causing the pituitary gland to secrete a hormone (prolactin) that is important for milk production. Another hormone from the pituitary's posterior lobe simultaneously affects the milk glands and ducts, causing the milk to be squeezed out of the breast. This hormone is called oxytocin and, via the blood, it also reaches the uterus, which contracts as well—something the mother can often feel at the beginning of a breastfeeding session.

In the first few days, her breasts are often swollen and tender. Initially, the breasts contain small quantities of what is called colostrum: this is particularly important for building up the newborn baby's immune system. After two or three days, the milk begins to flow. The sooner the mother puts the baby to the breast after birth, the easier it is to teach the baby to suck effectively.

All over the world, it is considered important to breastfeed babies during the first few months of life—and preferably longer—not only because it creates an intimate rapport between mother and child, but because mother's milk gives babies all the nourishment they need, and also excellent protection against infections. Though many healthy babies have been bottle-fed, and in some cases bottle-feeding may be necessary, the advantages of breastfeeding are clear and rewarding.

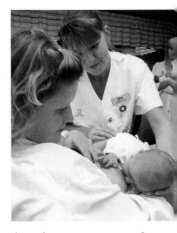

A newborn may nurse as often as 8–10 times a day, less frequently after the first few weeks. More nursing increases the milk supply.

Research has shown that, even if it is placed far down on the mother's stomach, the newborn baby can locate the breast within half an hour. The pictures *below* show the baby energetically struggling on and finally catching sight of the nipple. This instinct exists in animals and humans alike. But maternal assistance is welcome.

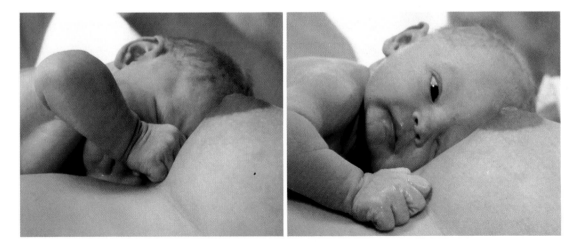

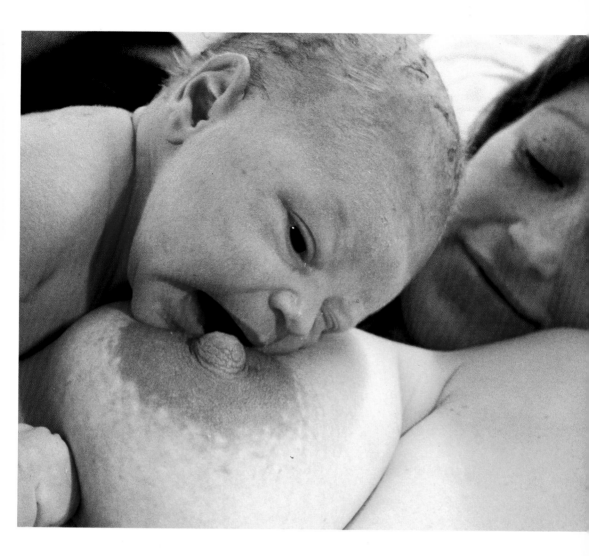

Breast is best

Breast milk contains all the
nutrients and minerals the
baby needs. Moreover, the
food is at the right temperature, and superior to any that
can be manufactured. There
are also strong emotional benefits; never again do the
mother and her baby have
such opportunities of getting
to know each other and forming a mutual attachment as
during breastfeeding.

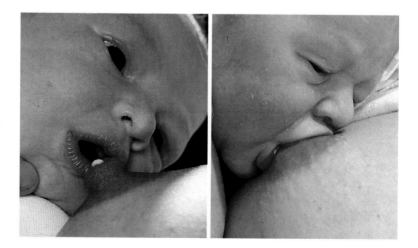

In the hospital

When all goes well, mother and baby are checked by a nurse—how the birth went, and whether anything in particular should be borne in mind—and then allowed to rest. In many hospitals, newborn babies remain in the same room as their mothers throughout the stay, in others, babies are placed in a nursery. During the hospital stay, midwives and nurses instruct and help the mother, and the father is also encouraged to take an active part.

The newborn baby needs a great deal of care and attention during the first few days; respiratory difficulty or irregular cardiac activity is not uncommon. Babies who show signs of being unwell may be sent to an intensive care nursery (called Special Care Baby Unit, SCBU, in the U.K.), or even to another hospital where specialized care is available.

After a normal delivery, the woman recuperates well within a few days. She spends a large part of the day with her baby. She may receive instruction from a physiotherapist concerning suitable exercises for the abdominal and pelvic muscles. She should start pelvic-floor contractions at an early stage. During the first few weeks, the stretched uterus bleeds, roughly as much as during menstruation or slightly less. In due course, the bleeding gives way to a brownish, then pinkish discharge for four or five weeks. The bleeding and the discharge are signs that healing is still taking place. The woman should consult with her doctor about bathing and intercourse. Contraception should be used as soon as intercourse resumes.

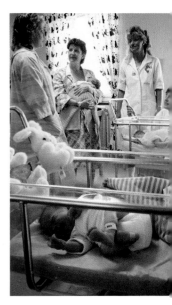

Giving birth is a major event in a woman's life, and the new mothers usually enjoy sharing their experiences with each other.

Older siblings may sometimes find it hard to understand why their mother devotes so much time to the newborn baby.

If it is her first child, the mother needs to practice looking after the tiny being.

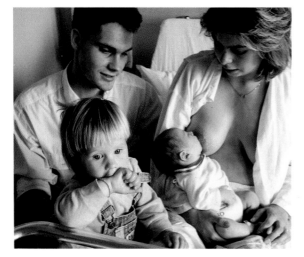

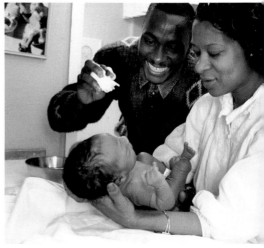

Back home

The new family goes home from two days to a week or so after birth, depending upon the well-being of mother and baby. By this time, newborns have been examined by a pediatrician, and may have regained their birth weight or at least started to put on weight after the initial loss. In the first few days, babies always lose a little weight, since the supply of food is relatively small and the intestines have not started to function properly.

Most babies are slightly sallow-complexioned, due to a chemical called *bilirubin* produced from the breakdown of red blood cells which are no longer needed in the new environment outside the uterus. If this sallowness is markedly yellow (neonatal jaundice), the baby is treated in the hospital during the first few days with special lights which break down bilirubin, and blood tests are repeated by the doctor for a certain period. Untreated jaundice of this kind may lead to brain damage in certain rare cases.

Coming home can be a stressful event, especially for first-time parents. Suddenly they have to bear the entire responsibility themselves. Feeding, changing and washing the baby take a long time, and in between most women need to rest. At night sleep is also severely disturbed at first by the baby's feedings—not to mention the fact that the mother is expected to cope with visits from relatives and friends. Most women do not feel that they have fully regained their strength until after five or six weeks.

Four to six weeks after delivery, parents usually take their

Before the journey home, the pediatrician checks all the baby's sensory and motor responses thoroughly. Walking reflexes are tested. A new mother usually has countless questions to ask.

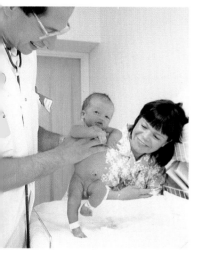

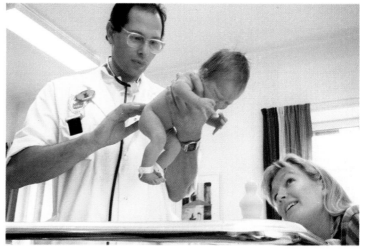

baby to the pediatrician or child health clinic for a first check-up. If problems arise before this, parents should call the doctor. In some areas, a visiting nurse will call on the family at home. In the U.K., this may be a health visitor or midwife.

Roughly six to eight weeks after birth, it is time for a last visit to the doctor. An internal examination with careful checks of the uterus and ovaries, and perhaps also cell samples from the cervix, is included in this consultation.

This is also a good time to decide on a suitable contraceptive. While nursing can delay the return of ovulation, this varies greatly and a reliable means of contraception is necessary as soon as a couple resumes intercourse. Another pregnancy following the first one too closely does not allow time to enjoy a period of discovery with the new baby and may be a severe strain on the mother.

After this visit to the doctor, the circle is complete: the woman has now experienced pregnancy, delivery and, not least, looking after a small new being—a member of the species that, without comparison in the animal kingdom, needs the longest period of support and assistance and most time for its development before it can stand on its own feet. The responsibility is enormous, and so is the joy.

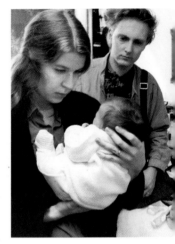

Home again! It feels wonderful, but at the same time a little frightening for parents to be on their own at home. At the hospital, there was help and expert advice at all times. Parents can visit the child health clinic—but still!

Below, Grandma has been in charge of the older children, and now she welcomes the littlest one home.

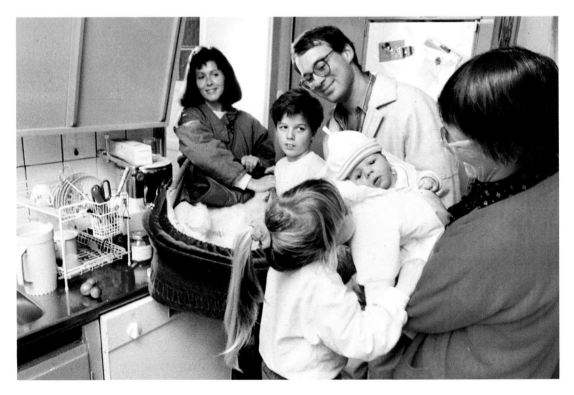

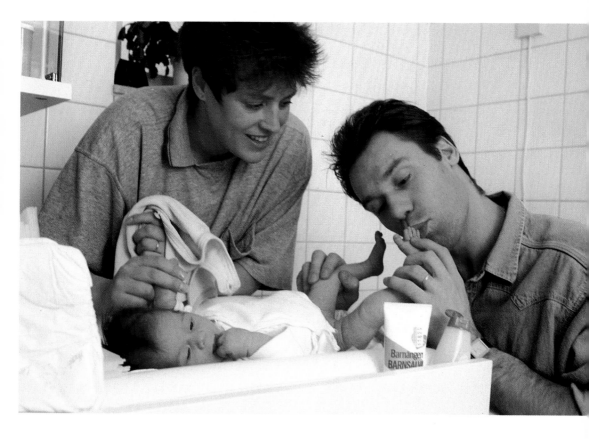

Everyday life begins

Despite all the support from childbirth education courses, the hospital, the pediatrician, relatives and friends, the new parents still feel uncertain when alone with their first-born. If he cries: why does he never stop? If he is not crying: has he stopped breathing? The mother wakes up at night at the slightest squeak or gurgle, and jumps out of bed to check.

Everyday life has begun, and having a baby in the house makes life completely different from the way it was before. What fantastic opportunities of growing and developing together with this tiny product of one's own flesh and blood!

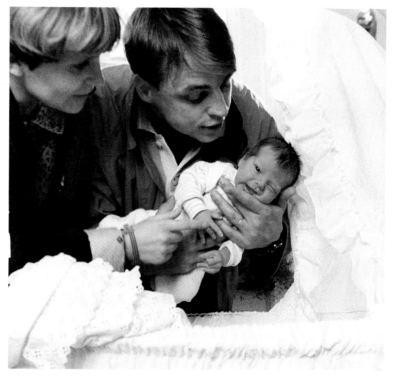

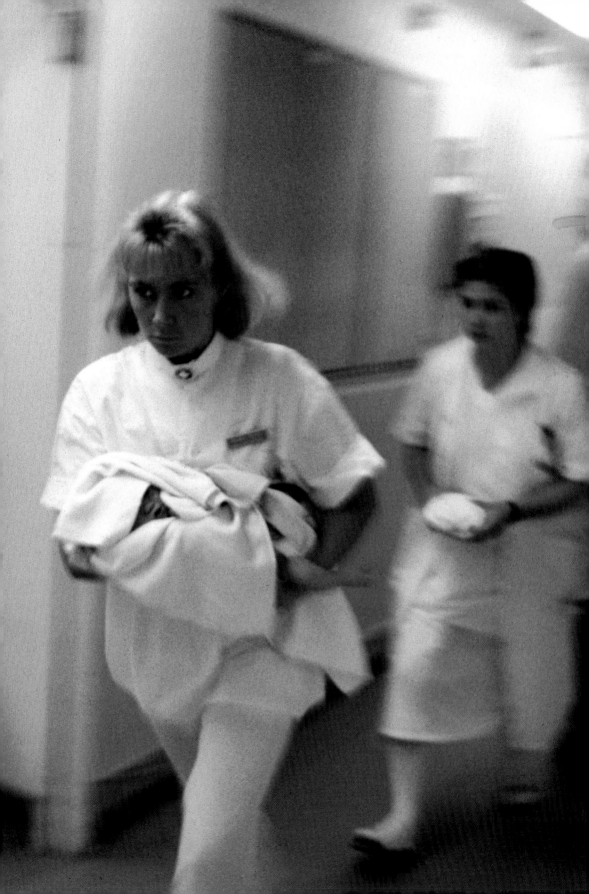

Special Care

So far, we have described pregnancy and delivery without complications, and this is indeed what happens in most cases. However, almost all expectant parents today know that pregnancy and childbirth also entail risks, primarily to the growing fetus, but also to the woman's health and life.

Early miscarriage is nature's way of preventing the further development of malformed fetuses. In certain countries, the woman can also opt—at least in early pregnancy—for an abortion if tests determine that a baby will be born with a severe defect or serious condition.

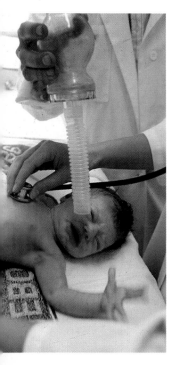

Sometimes, when a delivery is protracted and arduous for both mother and baby, the newborn baby must immediately be given extra oxygen. Soon its heart will beat normally.

After about the 24th week of pregnancy, a baby born prematurely has a chance of surviving and growing up without severe handicaps. Doctors who specialize in caring for premature babies have in recent years become more skillful, and gained access to increasingly sophisticated equipment. For women whose contractions start or membranes rupture prematurely, in particular, it is important to keep one's spirits up. Giving birth early no longer entails the same risk to the baby's health as it used to. The chances of the baby surviving and flourishing have increased enormously.

Obstetricians have also become more skillful at preventing premature labor. Early contractions, which are the commonest complication, are treated with bed rest, observation and pills or injections to relax the uterine muscles. Arresting the tendency toward premature labor for a few days often suffices, and both bed rest and medication may then be cautiously phased out.

Premature rupture of the membranes may be a more dangerous complication, since the risk of infection penetrating the uterus from the vagina is considerable. Nowadays, however, with rest and various antibiotic preparations, there is a good chance of all going well.

Twins, triplets, quadruplets, quintuplets—giving birth to more than one baby at the same time involves considerable risks of complications, and the more fetuses to be accommodated in the uterus, the greater these risks are. More than two babies at one birth is unusual when nature is left to take its course, but the increased use of pituitary-hormone treatment for certain types of infertility has boosted the incidence of multiple births. In a multiple pregnancy, the risk of not all the fetuses receiving an equally good supply of nutrients is relatively large, premature contractions and rupture of the membranes are relatively common, and even if the pregnancy proceeds until full term, the babies are usually smaller than when a single baby has had the uterus to itself.

Parents-to-be planning on delivery in a small local hospital should inform themselves ahead of time as to the nearest hospital equipped to care for high-risk newborns. The neonatal intensive care provided in large university hospitals (Special Care Baby Unit in the U.K.) can provide life-saving care for premature and other vulnerable babies.

Neonatal intensive care

Premature babies may have difficulty in using their lungs to absorb oxygen, and also their intestines for nutrient exchange. But with the stimuli of the outside world and careful nurturing,

The artificial uterus, the incubator, has—combined with many other technical refinements and advances in knowledge—helped to save the lives of many premature babies, enabling them to lead a normal life. Just a few years ago, they would not have had a chance.

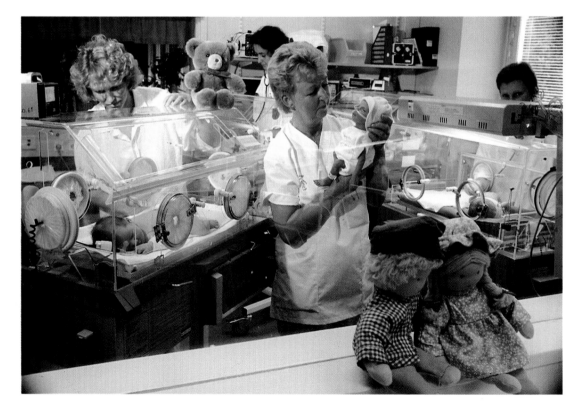

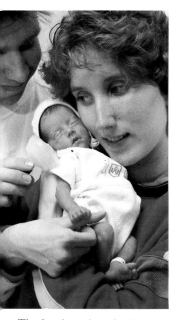

The family gathers for the first time. Such a tiny, fragile being! Holding one's baby is nevertheless a wondrous feeling.

most such babies rapidly mature and their essential motor and cognitive functions are satisfactory.

The fetus that has a severe handicap requires entirely different resources when it is born. Sometimes, emergency operations may be necessary within a day or two in order for the baby to survive; sometimes the pediatrician provides no active treatment, but simply monitors the baby's development. It is important that resources be available for rapid detection of defects or injuries to the heart, kidneys or intestinal tract of the newborn baby.

Some deformities that may seem alarming to the parents may, from the medical point of view, be quite commonplace. Cleft palate is one example. It is relatively common and can be repaired with good results by a skilled plastic surgeon. Hernias are also easily repaired.

Whether the problem is minor and easily corrected, or is irreversible or life-threatening, parents should insist on a complete explanation from the doctors. However small and handicapped a baby is, the parents' role is crucial. The mother and father must always remain close to the baby, and should also have repeated occasions for consulting pediatricians and nurses

After a few trying weeks, with raised blood pressure and marked swelling (edema), culminating in an acute cesarean section, the woman's feeling of shock gives way to the joy of having a live baby. *Right*, this baby weighed just over 700 g (about 1½ pounds) at birth. The mother is helping to look after her. The incubator provides an environment with the right temperature and the correct humidity (as high as 80 percent during the first week after birth). The respirator gives the baby additional help in breathing, and the heartbeat is monitored.

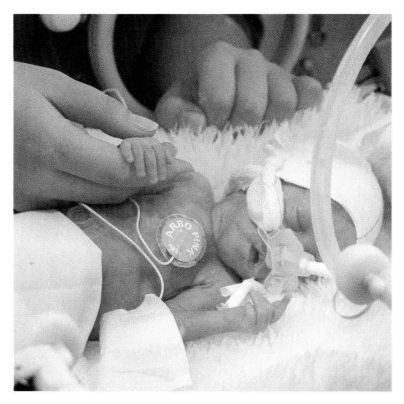

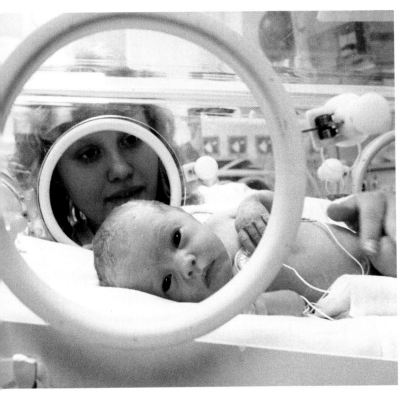

The days or weeks in the incubator must not become a period of isolation for the baby. Physical contact with the parents is of the utmost importance. Every infant needs caresses, hugs, skin contact and security.

The baby may benefit from being taken out of the incubator from time to time (*below*). The "kangaroo method," as it is called, enables parents to act in lieu of an incubator. The baby's respiration is aided by an upright position and by extra oxygen from the tube on the father's chest.

The mother can exercise the baby's sucking reflex by letting it practice at her breast at the same time as being tube-fed with milk that she has pumped out of her breasts in advance.

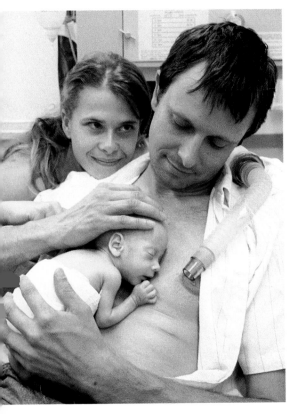

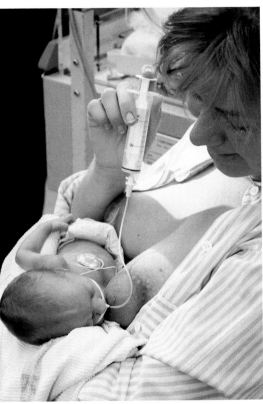

in the neonatal intensive care nursery (Special Care Baby Unit in the U.K.) about the child's development and the prognosis for the future.

These tiny or deformed children may need contact with the parents even more than others, in order to have the strength to survive their initial struggle. Learning to care for a baby with a low birth weight during the first few months, or one with an illness or handicap, requires considerable parental training and strong support from medical and nursing personnel of all categories.

Nevertheless, things do not always go well. The baby may die in the course of delivery, or within the ensuing week or month: the risk is not negligible. In statistical terms, it is not until a human being reaches the age of 70 or more that the mortality risk is as large as during the first week of life. Sometimes death is due to a severe, irreparable handicap, sometimes it cannot be explained. Research to prevent such tragic deaths and their causes is making important advances. Meanwhile, it is good to remember that more babies survive and grow up today than ever before in history.

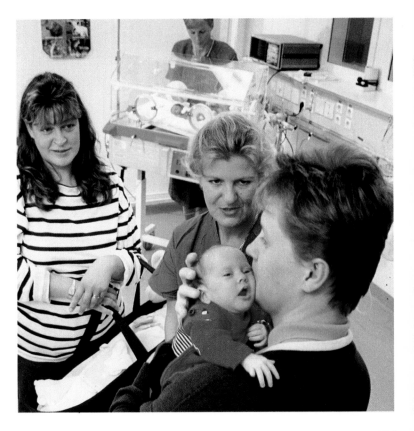

Time to go home! At last, these parents can take their baby home after its four-week stay in the neonatal intensive care unit.

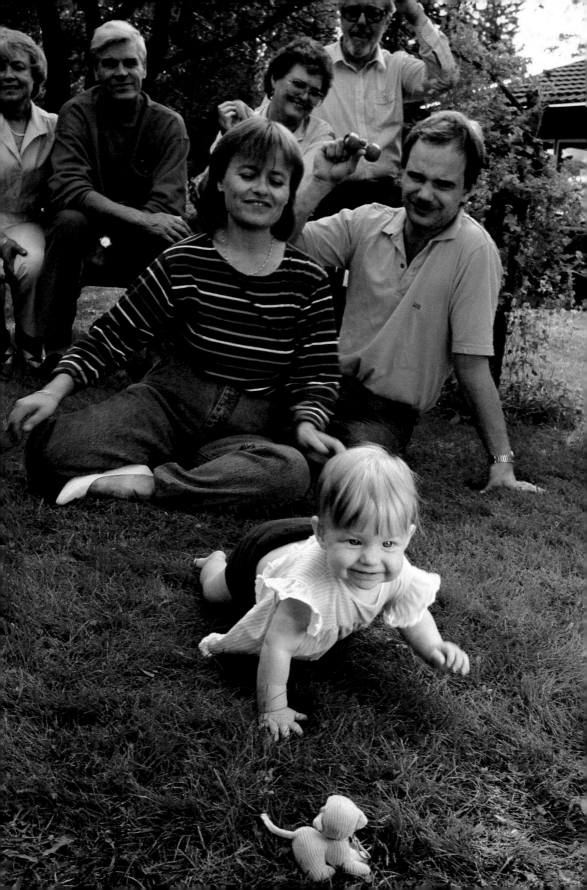

Our Genes

Why do we look as we do? Why are some of us tall, others short, some dark and others fair? How does a tiny embryo, with a tail like a seahorse, end up as a human being? The answers to these questions lie in our genetic code, which is unique to our species. As human beings, we differ greatly in our genetic characteristics. We cannot be confused with other species, nor can we reproduce outside our own species. This is a vital prerequisite of the development of species on Earth.

Although the human genetic blueprint is fixed, the wealth of variation is virtually infinite. There are no two people in the world with precisely the same genetic makeup, with the exception of identical twins, who—by definition—have exactly the same genes.

Within a single family, there are often certain similarities arising from the genes. Color of hair and eyes, height and a predisposition to a certain weight, state of health and longevity are more or less hereditary from one generation of a family to the next. Children often hear that they resemble their parents and grandparents. This is because half of the genes come from the mother and half from the father. Certain characteristics are usually said to be dominant (such as brown eyes), while others are recessive (blue eyes). For two brown-eyed parents to have a

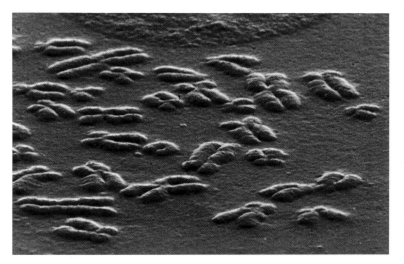

Three generations: the family inheritance lives on. Every cell of every individual contains the genes, with their coded hereditary blueprint that includes the ultimate secrets of life and has accompanied humankind throughout the millennia. This blueprint, which governs the individual's features down to the smallest detail, is expressed in a unique new combination in the new baby.

Right, some of the 46 human chromosomes that contain the genes.

blue-eyed child, each must carry the recessive gene for blue eyes. Where more complex mental characteristics are concerned, there may also be family similarities, but here upbringing and other external influences often play an important part. Thus, the genes leave scope for an individual to react to and be shaped by external influences. Without this possibility both upbringing and education would be somewhat meaningless.

Every cell in the human body has a nucleus, and the nucleus contains the genes. These do not form a shapeless mass, but in humans are located within 46 precisely shaped structures called chromosomes. All the cells in our body contain identical chromosomes, and by investigating a single cell of the human body, one can examine that individual's genes in detail.

The chromosomes bear DNA molecules, which constitute the actual memory of the cell. These are in the form of a long double helix on which coded chemical instructions are laid out. Each cell stores roughly 100,000 genes. These govern all the cell's functions and its reproduction, down to the tiniest detail.

Cells reproduce by division, whereupon two new cells arise with exactly the same genetic composition. Throughout the body, quantities of new cells that are exactly the same as the old ones are being formed every second. At the same time, many of the oldest cells are dying, and in this way our bodies keep themselves young and vigorous for a remarkably long time. Some cells, for example those of the brain and the ova in the ovaries, are incapable of dividing to form new cells, and we must therefore take extra care to help them to survive as long as possible.

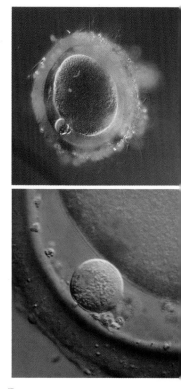

The hereditary blueprint for a human being is a theme with numerous variations in such characteristics as height, skin and eye color, sex, facial features and intelligence.

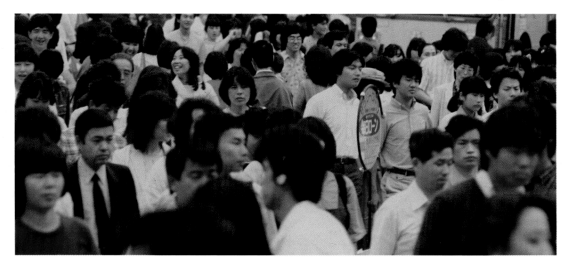

While ripening, the ovum halves its contingent of chromosomes to 23, relegating the surplus to the polar body, magnified *below left.* A similar splitting process takes place with sperm in the testicle (*below*). Each healthy sperm then contains 23 chromosomes, some of which are shown clearly here.

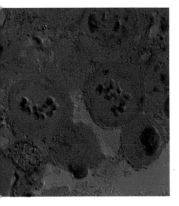

Below: the Y chromosome appears as a luminous white patch in three sperm heads. If one of these fertilizes the ovum, the baby will be male. The other five contain X chromosomes. *Right*, the sperm's 23 chromosomes, of which the Y chromosome (yellow) stands out with particular clarity.

Boy or girl?

The sex of a baby is determined when the sperm fertilizes the ovum. Twenty-three chromosomes from the mother and 23 from the father together provide all the genetic information needed for the new individual. The chromosomes form pairs, and the first 22 pairs are exactly the same, regardless of whether a boy or a girl has been conceived, while the 23rd pair indicates the sex of the fetus. In the female fetus, the 23rd pair comprises two X chromosomes, while in a boy it comprises one X chromosome and a smaller chromosome, called Y.

The course of events when the chromosomes of the sperm and the ovum merge is as follows: Normally, as we have seen, the human cell contains 46 chromosomes. The woman's ova has 46 chromosomes at the start, but when ovulation takes place and the ovum ripens, it discards half of its chromosomes. These are deposited outside the ovum and enclosed in a small sheath, where they form what is known as a polar body.

Similarly, the rudimentary sperm cells contain 46 chromosomes. Then, during the course of their development, the chromosomes separate, forming two identical sperm cells with 23 chromosomes each. One of the sperm formed in this way contains a Y chromosome, with the genetic basis for a boy, and the other an X chromosome that will result in a girl. When one sperm with its 23 chromosomes penetrates the ovum and unites with its supply of 23 more, the requisite 46 chromosomes are achieved.

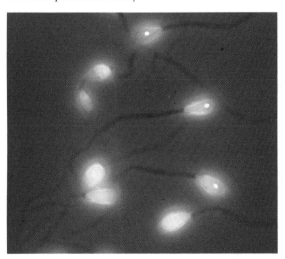

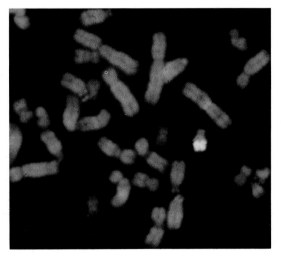

Amniocentesis

Sometimes the actual process of fertilization fails on the chromosomal level: the pairs of chromosomes do not connect, fragments of chromosomes break off, a piece of chromosome may become attached to another chromosome—the possibilities are numerous. In almost all cases, chromosome damage is so extensive and serious that the fetus cannot develop normally, and this results in an early miscarriage. Sometimes the chromosome damage is so limited as to be insignificant, but every so often the type of damage is somewhere between these two extremes, and a baby with deformities or illnesses may then be born. In order to detect such abnormalities, fetal genetic diag-

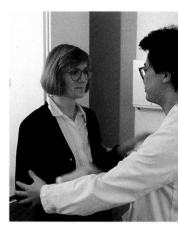

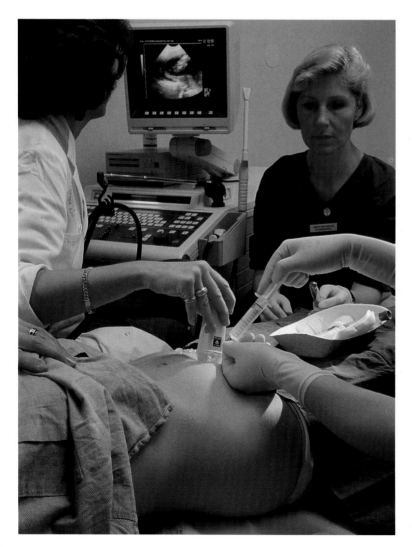

The amniotic fluid contains cells discarded from the fetus's skin, and these cells contain all the chromosomes. After the fetal position has been determined by means of ultrasound, the needle is inserted and the liquid withdrawn. The sample is shown to the mother (*right*) and sent to the laboratory, where the cells proliferate in a culture (*below right*).

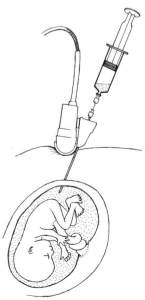

nosis is carried out more and more often. This entails the investigation and evaluation of the fetal chromosomes long before birth. These methods of chromosome analysis undeniably confer advantages, but can often raise difficult questions.

Amniocentesis carried out in the 16th or 17th week of pregnancy is the prevailing method at this time; it is based on the fact that fetal cells are released into the amniotic fluid. By means of a syringe and a long needle, a few milliliters of amniotic fluid are carefully withdrawn; after a few weeks' tissue culture, the chromosomes of the fetal cells can be examined to ensure that they are normal, allowing for the possibility of an abortion if they are not. The test also, of course, reveals whether the fetus is male or female, if the parents choose to know.

The chromosomes may be studied only when the cell divides. They are then photographed through a microscope and the negatives are enlarged, grouped and scrutinized. The chromosomes can reveal whether the fetus is carrying a hereditary disease.

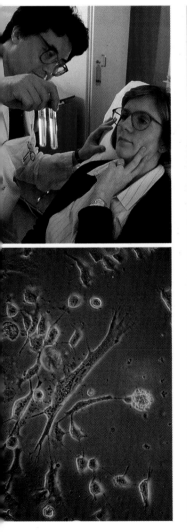

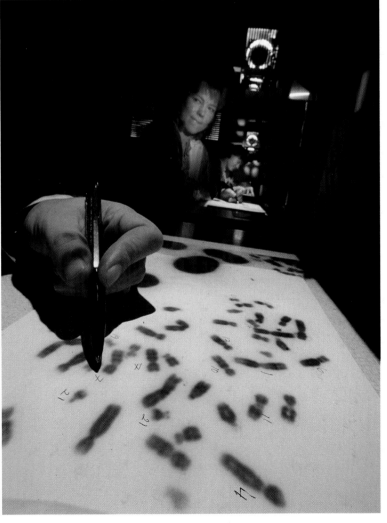

Earlier genetic diagnosis?

Regardless of the reason, a late abortion is always a major emotional trauma for the woman concerned, and in recent years, scientists have therefore begun to develop a method of chromosome analysis that may be used as early as the seventh or eighth week of pregnancy. This method is based on the removal by the obstetrician of a small piece of tissue from the chorionic villi, part of the placenta, which generally have the same chromosomal composition as the fetus. This method is known as CVS or chorionic villus sampling. Since more cells are obtained by this method than by amniocentesis, the chromosomal analysis may be completed within a day or so, and if chromosomal deviations are found, it is both psychologically and medically easier to carry out an abortion at this early stage. There is a small risk that the chromosomal composition of the cell sample may differ from that of the fetus, and that this form of analysis may therefore yield erroneous information and, perhaps, prompt an unnecessary abortion. In the future, in all probability, new and more accurate methods will become available.

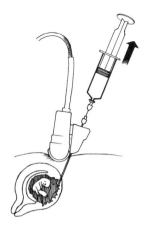

Chorionic villus sampling (CVS) is a new method whereby the obstetrician, using a needle, removes a small fragment of the placenta for testing. The sample contains chorionic villi, composed of countless tiny cells which generally contain the same chromosomal composition as the fetus.

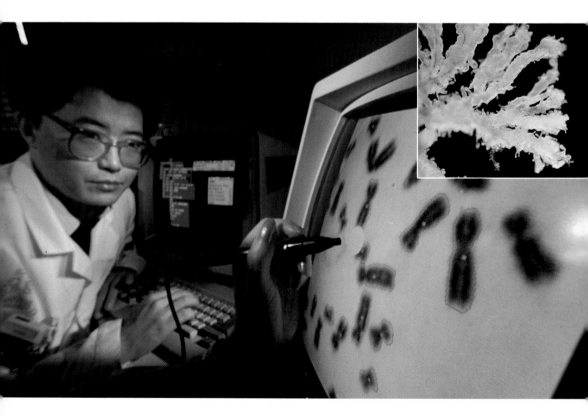

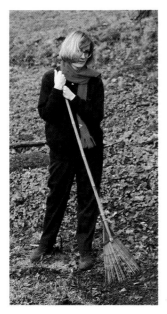

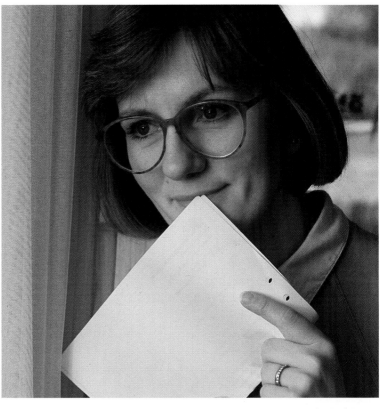

The wait for the result of amniocentesis is often both long and emotionally painful. This mother, who had previously given birth to a child with a grave genetic defect, had to wait several weeks.

An answer at last: the test was satisfactory and the fetus healthy. What joy! Now she can complete her pregnancy without worry.

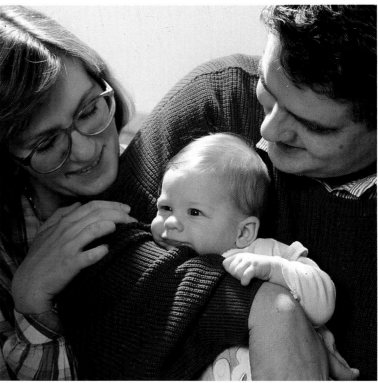

Right, the parents with their 7-month-old baby. Without fetal diagnosis, this couple might not have dared to bring another child into the world.

One chromosome too many

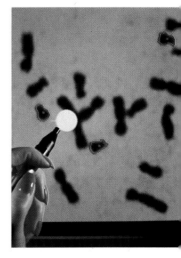

When chromosomal abnormalities are found by prenatal test-ing, a number of problems arise. Sometimes the deviation may be such that the doctors cannot definitely state to which abnor-malities it may possibly lead. Even if this can be predicted with a fairly high degree of probability, the woman may not wish to undergo a late abortion when she is confronted with the actual decision. Most mothers-to-be, in fact, assume that fetal diag-nosis is merely one extra check for safety's sake, and they have often not thought through, and worked out, how they may con-ceivably react if a chromosomal defect is definitely diagnosed.

In addition to chromosomal defects which arise at the time of fertilization or before, chromosomes and individual genes may, in the course of fetal development, incur defects, and the fetus is probably, in general, much more sensitive than the adult human being to such damage, known as a mutation. Radiation, toxic chemicals and air contaminants are among the causes of mutations.

The commonest chromosomal abnormality diagnosed is a defect in chromosome pair 21 whereby a third, extra chromo-some has been added to the pair ("trisomy," as it is called). This invariably results in Down syndrome. A child with Down syndrome thus has 47 chromosomes. The information from the extra chromosome enters into and affects the growth of the body, causing a series of external modifications that are easy to recognize: slanted eyes, malformed ears and abnormalities of the hands. These changes are accompanied by more serious internal abnormalities, often affecting the heart and always affecting intellectual capacity.

Down syndrome occurs more often when women become pregnant at a later age. The man's age is also thought to play some part. However, even a very young couple can produce a child with Down syndrome. Since it is relatively more common to become a parent at a young age, the majority of parents of children with Down syndrome are young, i.e. of an age at which genetic amniocentesis is not performed on a routine basis at this time.

The birth of a child with Down syndrome is a shock. Yet in families which face the challenge with love and understanding, both parents and siblings testify to positive experiences and the new dimension that such children can impart to life and the family.

Down syndrome

Down syndrome—named after the English doctor who described this handicap as long as 125 years ago—is caused by a surplus chromosome joined to chromosome pair 21. The phenomenon is called "trisomy" (*left*). The cause of this form of severe chromosome damage is unknown, but it has been established that older women are more often affected than younger ones.

These unusual children, while handicapped, can give parents and siblings a different attitude toward life and insight into its meaning. *Right*, two youngsters with Down syndrome who have found each other.

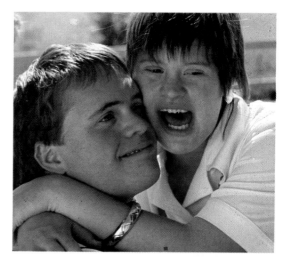

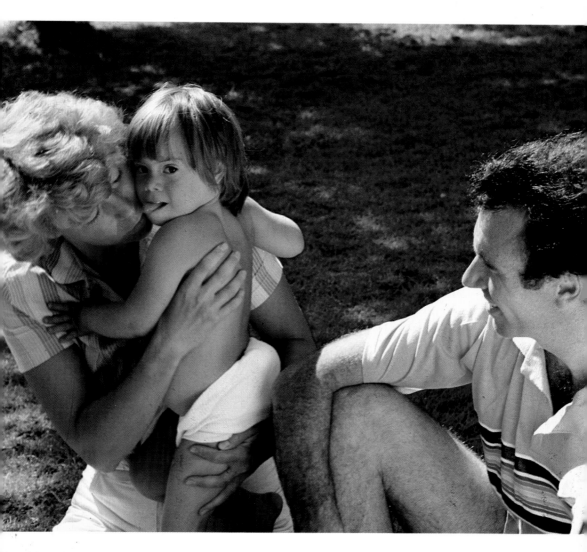

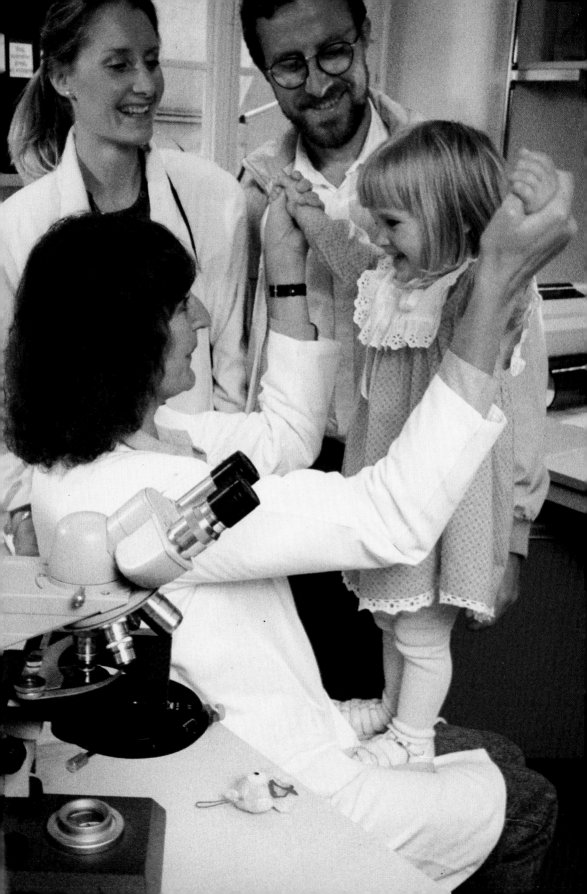

Difficulties in Conceiving

Between 10 and 20 percent of all couples are infertile. Exact statistics are hard to obtain, since we cannot easily distinguish between involuntary and voluntary childlessness. Numerous factors affect birth rates, such as political and religious attitudes, and economic conditions. Our external and internal environment, including such factors as environmental poisons and the stress of life in modern society, also affect our reproductive capacity.

When difficulties arise, both preventive and reconstructive measures are needed. Among the important tasks is that of informing people about, and treating, such "new" types of infection as herpes and chlamydia, which may impair human reproductive ability. The effects of certain contraceptives and especially of conditions in the workplace of both men and women need continuing research.

Is it, in general, a self-evident right of all human beings to produce children? Is infertility an illness or a handicap? Should society encourage and provide financial support to research on infertility? Should infertility treatment be provided free of charge and automatically at our hospitals? What are the ethical and legal problems in this context? The questions are innumer-

The team of skilled laboratory technicians and medical personnel involved in infertility clinics often become firm friends of the couples who have difficulty in conceiving. For this couple, the outcome was successful last time: a beautiful little girl. Now a second child would be most welcome.

Certain forms of infertility can be tackled by means of artificial insemination (*below*). The man's sperm are inserted in the uterus by means of a catheter. A period of intense waiting and hoping then follows.

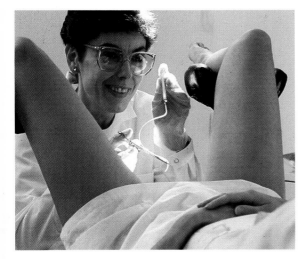

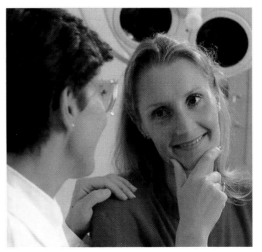

able, and to date largely unanswered. Nor are there yet any joint international rules or conventions providing guidance and answers to these questions, and meanwhile the explosive development of biological research constantly raises new and more difficult ones.

Globally, the population explosion is an enormous and threatening problem. The situation differs from country to country, however; Northern European countries, with very low birth rates, have put much emphasis on improved methods of treating infertility. The Chinese, who have problems of over-population, have reasons to pursue another policy (i.e. statutory family planning). Nevertheless, childlessness is an individual problem for each couple concerned, and can be just as hard to accept in China as anywhere else.

Since investigation and treatment are very expensive, they are in general confined to societies with adequate resources. However, according to recent reports, it is known that a major proportion of medical consultations in developing countries is occasioned by involuntary childlessness. In many of these countries, a large family is the parents' only insurance policy to provide for a secure old age.

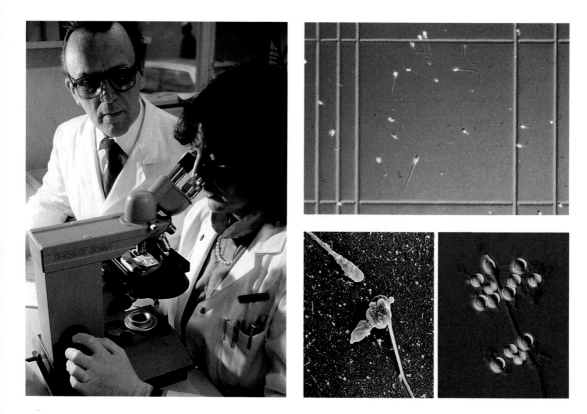

Treating male infertility

Considering various reasons for childlessness in purely medical terms, one may say, broadly speaking, that the cause lies solely in the woman in 40 percent of cases, solely in the man in 40 percent and in both sexes in 20 percent. Researchers have been most successful in treating female infertility, while options for helping infertile men have been very limited.

Fortunately, interest in male infertility and the potential for treating it have increased in the past few years. Improving the industrial environment is one vital preventive measure; preservation of sperm by freezing is another. When sperm counts are low, such methods as the insertion of sperm into the uterus, Fallopian tubes or even abdominal cavity may be feasible ways of facilitating the long journey through the cervix and uterus. *In vitro* ("test-tube") fertilization, too, requires far fewer sperm than fertilization resulting from sexual intercourse. The latest method to be investigated is the injection of a single sperm direct into the ovum. If this method proves possible to develop, very few men would be regarded as infertile.

How many sperm are there, and how mobile are they? Are many of them malformed? A microscopic examination of a fresh sperm sample provides answers to these questions. The sperm count is estimated by means of a grid. *Facing page, center, bottom row,* one healthy and one defective sperm.

The man may be allergic to his own sperm, and the woman may also be allergic to them. This can be ascertained by means of minute glass balls on which antibodies have been attached (*facing page, bottom right*). Medication or test-tube fertilization may sometimes help these couples.

Right insert, a swimming-speed test is performed on sperm in mucus from the cervix. *Right*, sperm and uterine mucus are combined for further microscopic tests.

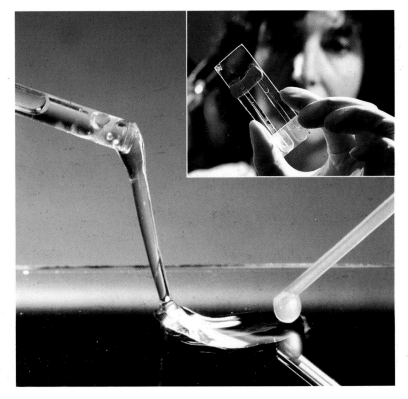

Hormonal treatment

One common cause of female infertility is hormonal imbalance. If this is sufficently disturbed, ovulation will fail to occur. Such a disturbance seldom reflects a serious illness but, untreated, leads to childlessness. The simplest form of treatment is a course of chlomiphene pills, given to the woman for five days shortly after her menstrual period begins. The treatment promotes the production of the hormones secreted by the pituitary gland, and this, in turn, affects hormone production in the ovaries, causing more follicles to ripen and rupture. The timing of ovulation, and thus the optimal time for conception, may be established almost to the hour by means of repeated hormone tests and ultrasound scans of the ovaries.

If the hormonal disturbance is more serious in nature, treatment with pills is inadequate. Instead, pituitary hormones are injected into the buttock muscles daily for a period of some ten days. This prompts ovulation in almost all cases, and the timing is determined in the same manner as with the pill treatment.

Multiple births can result from such treatments and couples should be aware of this possibility.

Are the Fallopian tubes open, enabling the ovum and sperm to meet? This can be checked by means of an X ray. Contrast fluid is sprayed in through the cervix, filling the uterus, and the X ray shows whether its passage through the Fallopian tube is unrestricted.

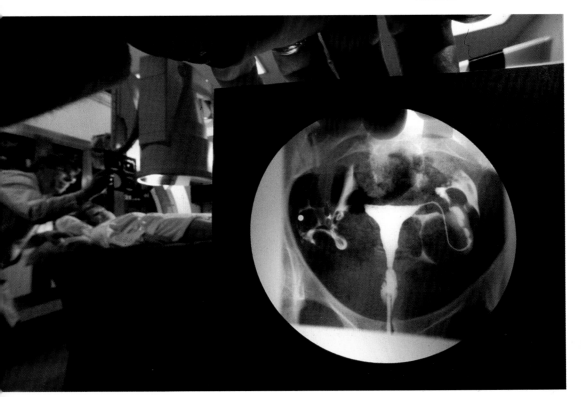

Microsurgery

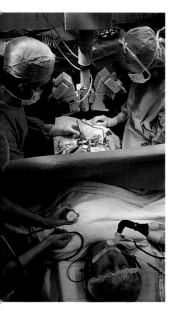

The microscope is a valuable aid to the surgical repair of damage to the Fallopian tubes caused by previous infections.

In order for hormonal treatment to succeed, the Fallopian tubes and uterus must be healthy, so that the ovum can be caught up by the Fallopian tube, be fertilized there and become implanted in the uterus. If the tubes are damaged—and this is a more frequent cause of female infertility than hormonal disturbances—efforts are usually made to repair the damage by surgical means. This operation requires considerable surgical skill and is carried out only at specialized hospitals or centers, using an operating microscope. Results vary, of course, depending on the extent of the damage, but on average one-third of the women who undergo it succeed in becoming pregnant.

Before the decision is taken to perform a microsurgical operation, both a contrast X ray and laparoscopy (an examination of the abdominal structures by means of an illuminated tubular instrument called a laparoscope) are, as a rule, carried out. Information from these investigations provides a basis for the operating procedure.

In recent years, *in vitro* fertilization has partially replaced microsurgery, or at least restricted its application. Surgery still undoubtedly has a part to play if the Fallopian tubes are only slightly damaged. Moreover, it yields the best results, and has the advantage that the woman can then have more children, since the outcome of the operation may last for many years.

One possible cause of the woman's infertility may be a constricted cervix, which can be dilated in a simple operation. But immunological infertility can also be a problem: the man's sperm react allergically against the cervical mucus or the mucous membrane's surface, rapidly losing their swimming capacity and perishing. This immunological reaction is usually a local one in the cervix, and if the sperm are put straight into the uterus, this problem can sometimes be overcome.

What joy! After years of involuntary childlessness, the woman has been treated successfully: she is now pregnant. And the doctor gets a hug.

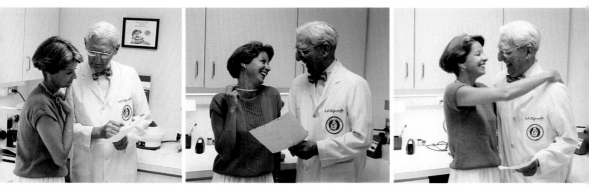

197

Fertilization outside the body

One new method of treating certain forms of both female and male infertility is fertilization outside the body (*in vitro* or test-tube fertilization). In the 1980s, the method became widespread: during that decade, more than 25,000 babies were born worldwide thanks to this technique.

The first "test-tube baby" was born in Britain in 1978, thanks to the work of the British doctors Robert Edwards and Patrick Steptoe. However, the concept is a very old one. As early as 1890, August Strindberg described with almost uncanny foresight, in a short-story collection entitled *By the Open Sea*, how the narrator obtains a human ovum and studies it under a microscope, after enclosing it in an incubator with a temperature of 36°–41° C (about 96°–105° F). He adds sperm and watches proudly how they move and fertilize the ovum, which then starts to divide.

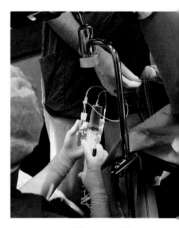

Aspiration of the ova. The woman lies, fully conscious, on the operating table as for a pelvic examination. The gynecologist uses ultrasound to guide the insertion of a needle toward the ovarian follicle via the vagina, which is locally anesthetized. By means of suction, the contents of the follicle are withdrawn into a test tube.

Test-tube fertilization today takes place as follows: One or more ova are removed from the woman's ovaries on the estimated ovulation date. The ova are placed in a nutrient solution kept at 37° C (98.6° F). After a few hours, a small quantity of sperm from the man is added, and the ova and sperm are left to fuse for 24 hours or so. The ovum is then placed in a new culture medium, inspected under the microscope and then incubated for another day or so. Thus, the process that has always happened far inside the woman's Fallopian tube now can take place in a laboratory. If fertilization has occurred—as it does in four cases out of five—the ovum has now divided into two to six cells and is ready to be carefully implanted in the woman's body. Through the vagina and cervix, the fertilized ovum is introduced into the uterus by means of a thin plastic cannula. Rates of success vary from one institution to another; roughly 10 to 20 percent result in a full-term pregnancy.

One method of treating *inexplicable infertility* has been dubbed GIFT. Naturally, the American researchers pioneering the method had in mind the everyday sense of the acronym, but GIFT is in fact an abbreviation for "Gamete Intra Fallopian Transfer." In brief, the method is based on the aspiration of one or more ova from the ovaries and their immediate transfer to the Fallopian tube, along with sperm from the man. This method results in pregnancy in some 30 percent of cases, but it should be noted that it is feasible only if the woman's Fallopian tubes are functioning normally and is therefore no alternative to test-tube fertilization.

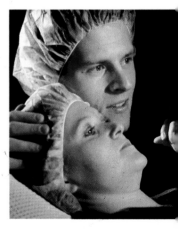

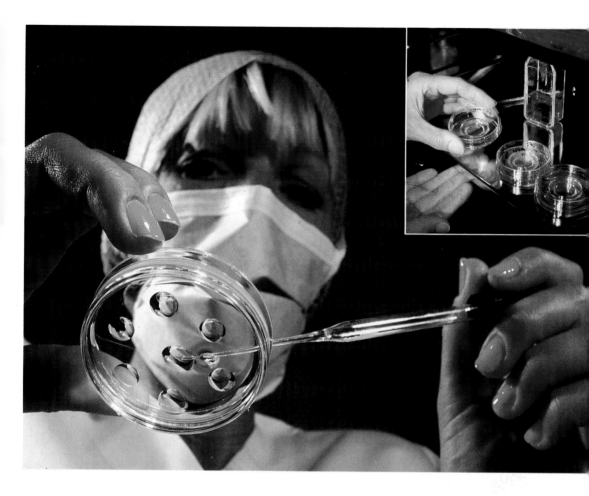

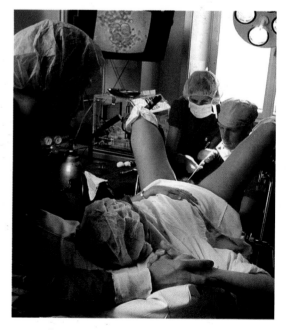

Helping nature

In certain forms of infertility, the ripe ovum must be removed from the woman's body to be fertilized. The pictures on these pages show how a "test-tube baby" is conceived.

Top left, we see how one or more ova are aspirated from the ovary at the time of ovulation. *Above*, seven ova in a glass bowl surrounded by nutrient solution. The sperm are added with a pipette. The ova and sperm are then placed in a warm container, an incubator, in which the temperature and air humidity are subject to careful control.

Two days later, the ovum fertilized in this way has divided and now comprises two to six cells. With a thin plastic cannula, one or more fertilized ova are gently inserted into the uterus. In roughly one-fifth of cases, the procedure culminates in pregnancy. If it fails, new attempts can be made with the remaining fertilized—and deep-frozen—ova.

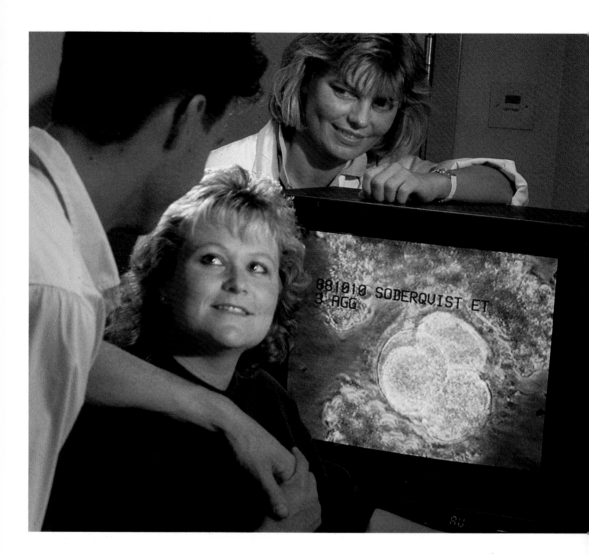

Insert, right: the fertilized ovum is inserted with a thin plastic cannula into the woman's body, and placed at the summit of the uterus. The pale patch is the opening of the Fallopian tube.

Right, the fertilized egg has settled on the endometrium and is being transformed into a blastocyst, which becomes firmly anchored to the membrane, constructs a placenta and in due course develops into an embryo, a fetus, and a baby.

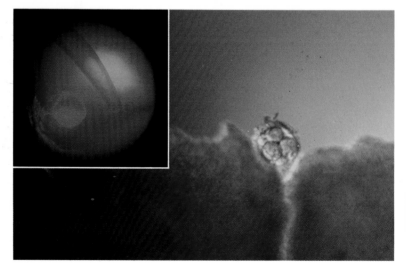

Two portraits of one baby

The ovum has divided! *Left*, the nurse shows the hopeful parents an enlarged image of their own fertilized ovum immediately before insertion into the woman's uterus. The ovum has been cultured for two days in a nutrient solution, and has now divided into four cells.

In this case, the joint efforts of the parents and the research team succeeded: the woman conceived, and the couple rejoice that they will soon have a baby of their own.

Below, the proud parents afterward with their own, longed-for baby. It is astonishing, and almost impossible to grasp, that the baby has developed from the four cells on the screen.

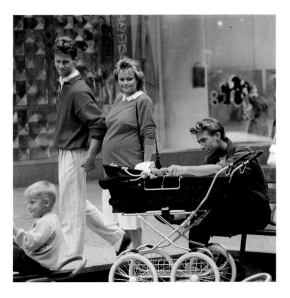

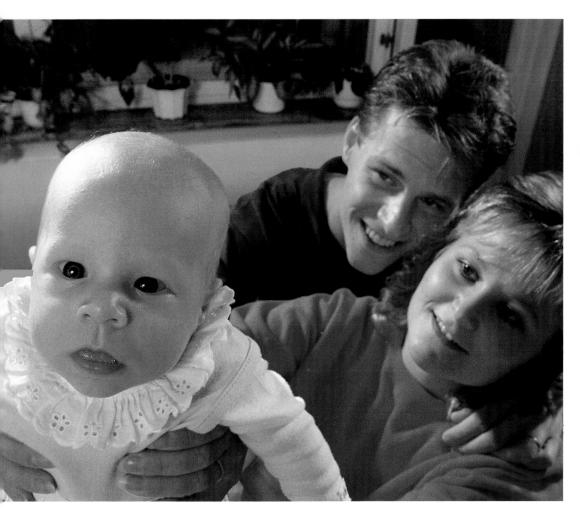

Research in human reproduction

Developments in this field—as in so many others—are taking place at such a breakneck speed that a large number of what we now regard as future opportunities will be utilized in our hospitals within only a few years.

Deep-freezing of sperm at an ultra-low temperature (–196° C), using liquid nitrogen, is one method of keeping the sperm viable over long periods. After careful thawing, the sperm once more start moving, and they retain their capacity to fertilize ova. This method has been used for the past decade or so in many parts of the world, often for men with tumors in their testicles, where surgery or chemotherapy will destroy the sperm. It has been suggested as an option for men in certain hazardous industries, where there is a danger of toxic chemicals gradually impairing their sperm and fertility. Obviously, such an indirect solution to a dangerous workplace is controversial.

Deep-freezing of unfertilized ova has proved to be considerably more difficult, and only a few attempts culminating in successful pregnancies have been made.

Freezing of fertilized ova, on the other hand, is simpler, and several thousand babies have already been born after the fertilized ova from which they developed had been frozen at various stages of development and subsequently thawed. Why is this technique used? The primary reason is that *in vitro* fertilization sometimes gives rise to numerous fertilized ova at a single attempt. Quite simply, not all the ova can be inserted in the uterus, since the risk of triplets and quadruplets would be too great. The fertilized ova may then be frozen and preserved for a few months, and if the woman has not become pregnant on the first occasion, the frozen ova may be used. Another option may be to keep the fertilized ova for a future pregnancy if the woman has conceived at the first attempt.

Experiments involving the *injection of sperm into the ovum* have already been carried out successfully, and this is a method that could assume importance for men with almost immobile sperm or a low sperm count. A sperm sample from an ejaculation containing less than five million sperm cannot, in general, give rise to pregnancy as a result of normal intercourse. In fertilization outside the body, some 10,000— 100,000 sperm may suffice, but with the new injection method, only a few are required.

In the future, it will also be possible to utilize the fertilized ovum's distinctive properties in various ways by means of *embryo diagnosis*. This is because the cells of a fertilized ovum are

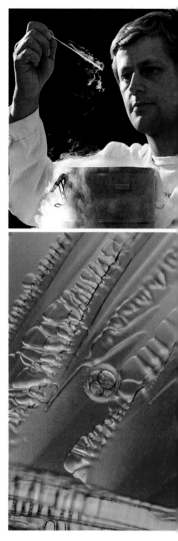

Sperm and fertilized ova can be preserved by deep-freezing for long periods, in liquid nitrogen (at –196° C; about –321° F). If thawed gently, they can regain their vital processes after their long slumber. The ice crystals surrounding the fertilized ovum melt slowly.

characterized, during the first few divisions, by what is known as totipotence (toti = complete; potence = capacity), i.e. each cell has the ability to convey the entire human genetic blueprint. Some of the cells may, without any damage to the embryo, be used for chromosomal analysis or sex determination. Such experiments have already been carried out on human ova, and could become very important for couples carrying some known hereditary disease that affects only one sex. It would then be possible to ensure that the fertilized ova introduced into the uterus have normal chromosomes, and thus to avoid abortions prompted by the diagnosis of impairment at a much later stage by means of conventional amniocentesis.

On the subject of the future of reproduction, we should, finally, make some mention of opportunities for improving fetal prospects during pregnancy, using *fetal surgery*. The fetus, in common with the growing or adult human being, may incur illnesses or injuries that can be alleviated or cured. Improved and accurate techniques of fetal diagnosis, by laboratory tests, ultrasound and other means, can tell us that the health or life of a fetus inside the uterus is in jeopardy.

Microinjection of the sperm direct into the ovum. This method of the future may be highly significant for men with few sperm, or sperm of poor mobility. We see a sperm in the needle being inserted through the ovum wall. Dimensions: the ovum measures 0.1 mm (about .04 inch) and the sperm 0.06 mm (about .024 inch) in length.

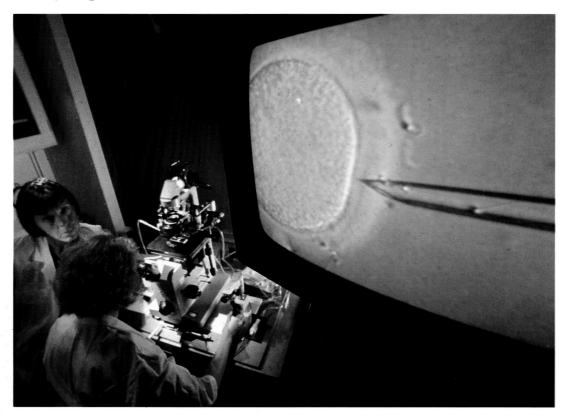

Fetal anemia arising from Rh immunization is one example of a disease that is medically curable today: using mobile ultrasound images, doctors insert catheters and give the fetus blood transfusions. Certain kidney injuries may be diagnosed at an early stage, and catheters can relieve the kidneys. A case of hydrocephalus may be diagnosed early and sometimes treated by certain intrauterine operations to prevent severe brain damage. Cardiac surgeons believe that, in the near future, it will be possible to intervene before birth and remedy certain types of grave cardiac defect as early as at the fetal stage. The methods abound, and they are all aimed at improving the fetus's chances of developing normally and, after birth, leading a life that is as meaningful as possible.

However, all these methods and options also impose severe psychological strains on the parents of today and tomorrow. Must we really use all these advances of modern science? Cannot pregnancy and birth remain "natural" and not manipulated by technology? Cannot we, as parents, place our faith in everything going as it should? Individual views on these matters must be respected, and it goes without saying that all staff at maternity clinics and hospitals who come into contact with a pregnant woman and her partner must pay attention to the couple's worries and preoccupations, and always seek to understand their innermost wishes.

Finally, let us remember that pregnancy is not an illness. It is the most stupendous life process that we undergo, and the biological selection strategies of millennia have made human reproduction ever more perfectly adapted to its purpose.

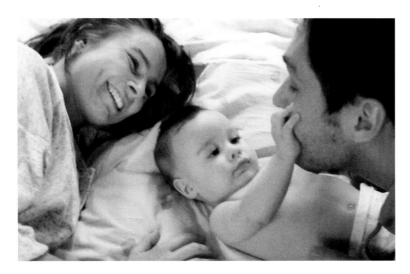

Tiny and powerful — the very helplessness of newborn babies is perhaps their greatest strength. They awaken deep emotions in us and create enduring attachments.

Having a baby in a world with five billion human inhabitants — a world that is undergoing a population explosion — is, in one sense, the most everyday of events. But for the woman who has nurtured and borne the baby it is something else. Giving birth is nothing short of a miracle: the greatest miracle in her life.

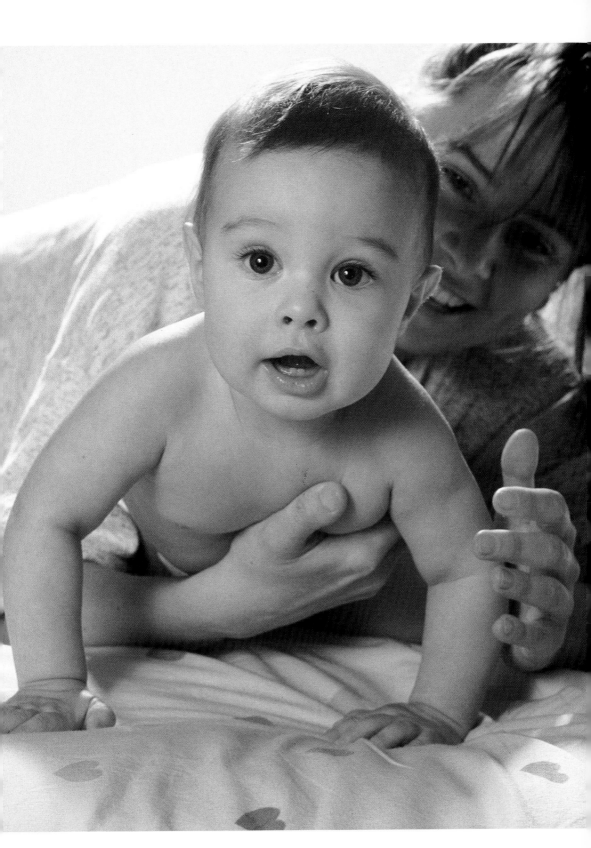

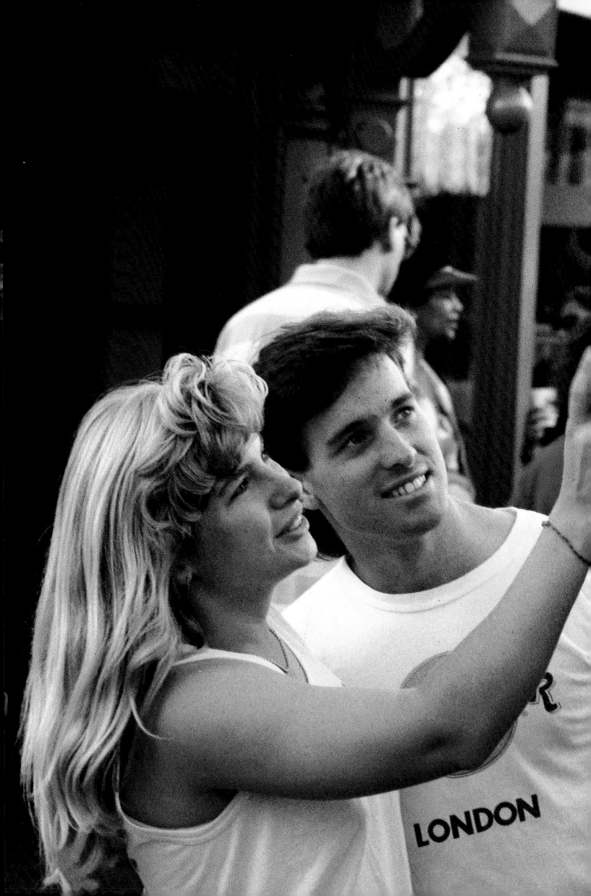

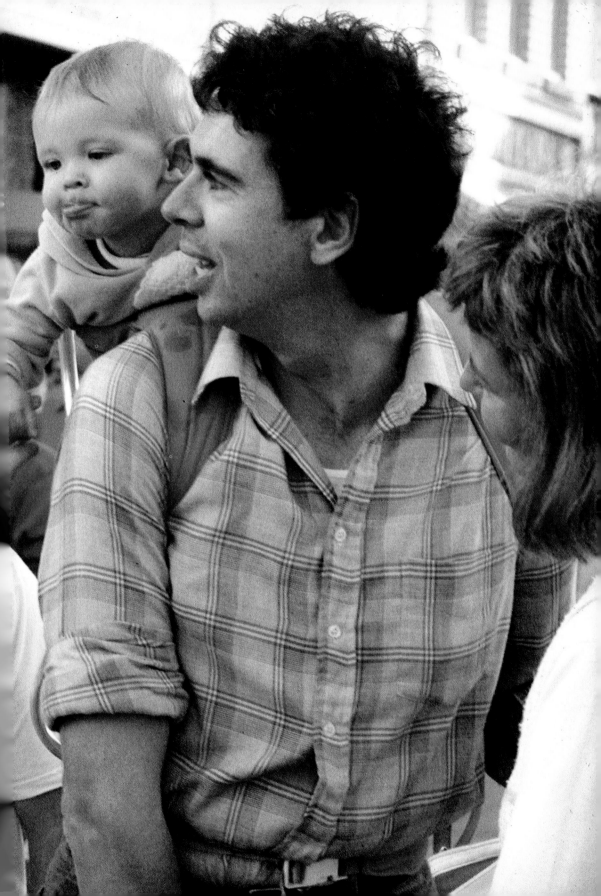

Acknowledgments

This book is the result of cooperation between a large number of people. A particularly important contribution has been that of a small group of close colleagues who, in various ways, have continuously provided ideas and advice in the course of many years' work. Warm thanks are due to Bo Berling, Ebbe Carlsson, Anne Fjellström, Thomas Fjellström, Lars Hamberger, Svend Lindenberg, Anita Sjögren, Hanne Tinggaard and Per Wivall.

For all her love, encouragement and help in creating this book, I would also like to thank my wife Catharina.

Heartfelt thanks, too, to all the couples who have shown great trust in allowing me to be present at, and take photographs of, the very private moment when their child was born. And warm thanks to the obstetric staff who let me and my assistant work alongside them.

Lennart Nilsson

A large number of researchers, doctors, technicians and hospital staff have provided invaluable help in the creation of this book. Not all of them can be mentioned by name here, but the photographer, the author and the publisher alike would like to thank them all warmly for their great goodwill and complaisance.

Conception, implantation and in vitro fertilization: Prof. Grete Byskov, Dr Svend Lindenberg and laboratory assistant Hanne Tinggaard, the Copenhagen National Hospital; university secretary Ann-Louise Dahl, Prof. Lars Hamberger, Prof. Per Olof Janson, Peter Sjöblom, Ph.D. and licentiate Anita Sjögren of the Gynecological Clinic at Sahlgrenska Hospital, Gothenburg; laboratory assistant Anita Peura of the Monash Medical Centre, Melbourne, Australia; Dr The-Hung Bui, Prof. Marc Bygdeman, Dr György Csemiczky, registered midwife (RM) Maria Edler, laboratory engineer Marita Johansson, RM Gunilla Landberg, RM Anita Malmgren and Assoc. Prof. Håkan Wramsby of the Gynecological Clinic at Karolinska Hospital, Stockholm; Assoc. Prof. Örjan Lundqvist and Dr Måns Palmstierna of the Gynecological Clinic at Akademiska Hospital, Uppsala; and Assoc. Prof. Lars Marsk and Assoc. Prof. K.G. Nygren, RM Margareta Stefansson, Assoc. Prof. Peter Svallander and laboratory assistant Anne-Marie Thörnblad of the IVF unit at Sophiahemmet Hospital, Stockholm.

Male reproductive physiology: Prof. Leif Plöen, Dept. of Anatomy and Histology, Faculty of Veterinary Medicine, SLU, Uppsala; Prof. Lennart Andersson, Urological Clinic, Karolinska Hospital; Assoc. Prof. Ulrik Kvist and laboratory assistant Inger Söderlund, Andrology Section, Karolinska Hospital; Assoc. Prof. Bengt Fredricsson of the Andrological Unit, Gynecological Clinic, Huddinge Hospital; Assoc. Prof. Rune Eliasson and Assoc. Prof. Öivind Johnsen of the Dept. of Reproductive Physiology, Karolinska Institute; RM Marie Antonsson, Assoc. Prof. Rune Eliasson, Assoc. Prof. Staffan Norén and laboratory assistant Eva Örn of the Andrological Unit at Sophiahemmet Hospital.

Maternity and child care: RM Eivor Björkman and Dr Lena Lagerström-Lindberg of Zinkensdamm maternity clinic, Stockholm, and RM Gunilla Primén of the Maternity Clinic at Danderyd Hospital, for their editorial revision; and the staff of several other maternity clinics in Stockholm and maternity wards at Karolinska Hospital and Söder Hospital.

Ultrasound: RM Gunilla Landberg, Assoc. Prof. Harry Lindholm, registered general nurse (RGN) Ella Söderlind and RM Britt Trygg-Hemmingsson of the Gynecological Clinic, Karolinska Hospital.

The baby's nutritional absorption: Assoc. Prof. Olle Björk and Prof. Hugo Lagercrantz, Child Health Clinic, Karolinska Hospital.

Photography using magnetic resonance: X-ray assistant Elna Berglind, Dr Håkan Göransson and Assoc. Prof. Tomas Hindmarch of the Dept. for Magnetic Resonance Imaging, Karolinska Hospital.

Delivery: RM Gudrun Abascal of the Obstetric Ward at Danderyd Hospital, for editorial revision, and also the staff of the obstetric wards at Nacka, Karolinska, Huddinge, Söder and Sahlgrenska Hospitals.

The newborn baby's imitation capacity: Dr Carin Holmlund, Dept. of Education, Stockholm University.

Premature babies: the neonatal wards at Danderyd and Karolinska Hospitals, Stockholm, and Sahlgrenska Hospital, Gothenburg.

Chromosome investigation and DNA analysis: Assoc. Prof. Lennart Nilsson of the Dept. of Physiology, Karolinska Institute, and Prof. Jan Lindsten of the Clinical Genetic Laboratory at Karolinska Hospital.

Valuable help with operation pictures: RGN Sonja Ekelund, Dr Jonas Harlin and RGN Inga Nilsson of the Central Surgery Dept., Karolinska Hospital; RGN Eva Andersson, Dr Lena Granström, Dr Margareta Nyman, Dr Henrik Rabaeus and Dr Kerstin Wersäll of the Surgery Dept. at Danderyd Hospital; RGN Kerstin Bourdin, Dr Einar Pálsson and Dr Sven Olov Sandström of the Surgery Dept. at Nacka Hospital; Dr Jane Andersson, Assoc. Prof. Bo A. Nilsson, RGN Ingmarie Norström, Dr Ulla Roth-Brandel and RGN Anna Lisa Wiberg of the Surgery Dept. at the Gynecological Clinic, Söder Hospital.

Help with English translation: Dr John Yeh, Dept. of Obstetrics and Gynecology, Harvard Medical School, Boston, USA.

Valuable technical information: Prof. Gunnar Bergström of the Dept. of Chemical Ecology, Gothenburg University; Prof. Elisabeth Johannisson of WHO, Geneva.

Special thanks to: Professors Howard and Georganna Jones of the Institute for Reproductive Medicine, Norfolk, USA; Northic General Hospital, Norfolk, USA; Prof. Robert Edwards of the University of Cambridge, UK; Prof. Antonin Zwinger, Dr Jana Jedliekova, Assoc. Prof. Jan Jirasék and Dr Pavel Smeral of the Research Institute for the Care of Mother and Child, Prague; Dr Chan Kong Hon and Dr Mary Rauff of Kandang Kerbau Hospital, Singapore; Dr S. Arulkumaran of the National University Hospital in Singapore; Dr Tjokorda Gde Subamia at the Kuta Health Centre, Bali; the Swedish Broadcasting Company; and the Swedish Medical Research Council.

Technical information

Manufacture of special optics: graduate engineers Georg Vogel, Stockholm, and Bo Möller, Zeiss, Oberkochen, West Germany.
Custom-made endoscopes: Karl Storz GmbH, West Germany.
Development and manufacture of the scanning electron microscope: Jeol, Tokyo, Japan.
Manufacture of photographic aids: Steen and Erik Lorentzen, Lorentzen Instrument AB.
Microscope equipment: Nikon.
Image analysis of fluorescence microscopy: Dr Michael Cohn, AB Parameter.
Thermocamera: engineer Jan-Åke Andersson, Agema Infrared System AB.
Magnetic resonance image on page 147: X-ray assistant Elna Berglind, Karolinska Hospital.
Electron-microscopic preparation technique: Prof. K. Tanaka, University of Tottori, Japan.
Electron-microscope expert: Lauri Saastamoinen, Jeol Skandinaviska AB.
Light-microscope experts: Åke Brunkener, Sven Bådholm, Gabriel Marx, Zeiss.
Technical assistance: engineer Björn Holmstedt, Immuno Sweden AB; Assoc. Prof. Masaya Takumida, Hiroshima, Japan; laboratory assistant Anne Marie Lundberg of the research unit at the Ear, Nose and Throat Clinic, Karolinska Hospital; Dr Kristina Sundqvist of the Dept. of Toxicology, Karolinska Hospital.
Photographic assistants: Anne Fjellström, Thomas Fjellström and Niklas Dahlskog.

To enhance clarity in pictures taken with the scanning electron microscope, these have been artificially colored using a special method – converting shades of gray into colors by means of separation – developed by photographer Gillis Häägg, Gothenburg.

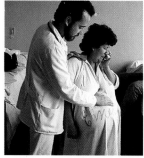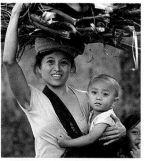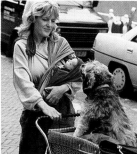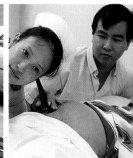
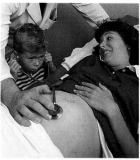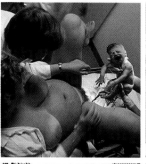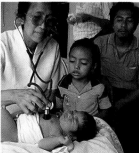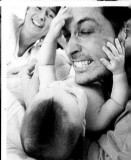
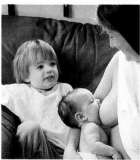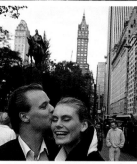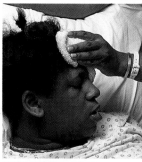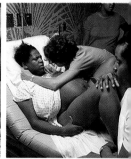
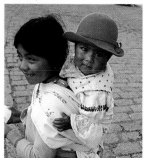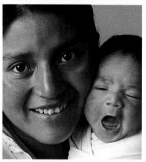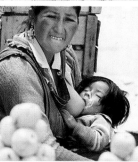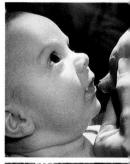
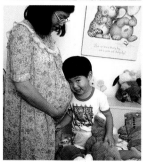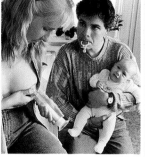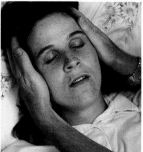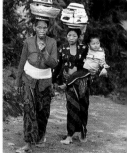

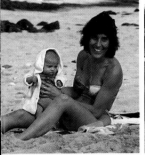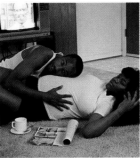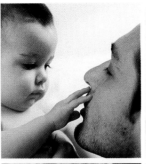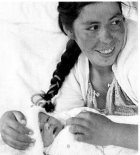
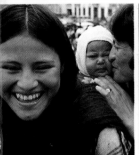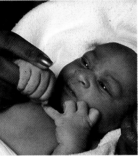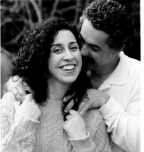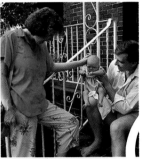
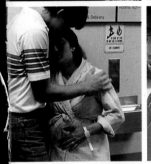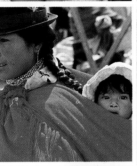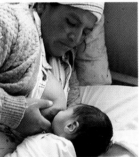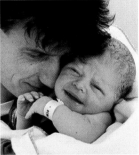
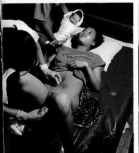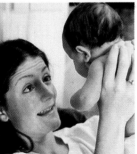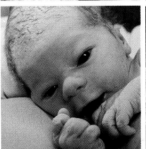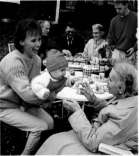
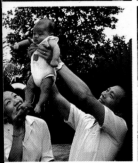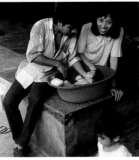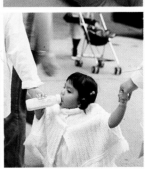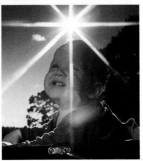

Index

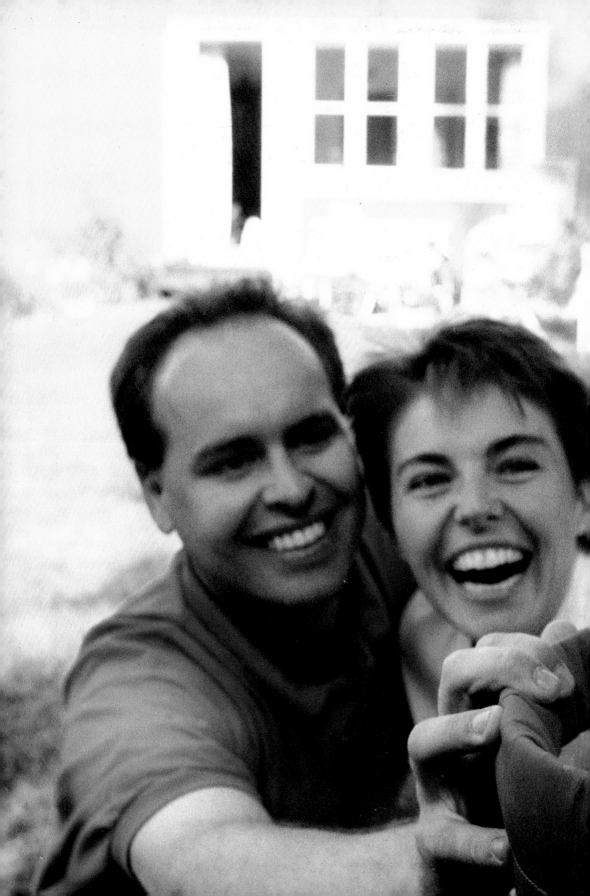